your
ACTION
potential

your
ACTION
potential

Dr. Jonathan Yalowchuk

TATE PUBLISHING & Enterprises

Published by Tate Publishing & Enterprises, LLC
127 E. Trade Center Terrace | Mustang, Oklahoma 73064 USA
1.888.361.9473 | www.tatepublishing.com

Tate Publishing is committed to excellence in the publishing industry. The company reflects the philosophy established by the founders, based on Psalm 68:11,
"The Lord gave the word and great was the company of those who published it."

Published in the United States of America

ISBN: 978-1-60799-246-2
1. Health & Fitness / Naprapathy
2. Medical / Alternative Medicine
09.08.10

Dedication

I would like to dedicate this book to a very special someone who has had such a profound effect on my life and me and continues to do so even though he is no longer of this earth. He steered me toward knowledge kicking and screaming, without any idea that my eventual destiny would be to become a "doctor," translation teacher, to share the gift that he gave me in one form or another. Words can never explain the magnitude of what he gave to me and the lessons he instilled on my soul. He made me understand that I could do anything I wanted to do in life. "You just have to act and the rest will fall into place." The universe produces very few people like Mr. Harold B. Morris. I am just honored that I got to share his time while he was here. You are loved and missed from the bottom of my heart.

Acknowledgments

This could be long and drawn out, and I will do my best to make it as concise as possible. I would like to thank all my friends, you know who you are, for being there in thick and thin; it is a gift to have you in my life.

To my family, as a whole, for all your love and support, without you I would not know where I would be. I feel that my life could be very different now.

To my sisters, for all their love and protection. It helps to have a cheering section and also someone to let you know when you were getting out of line. To my niece and nephews, I am so proud of you guys.

Joshua, I can not wait to present you with your diploma when you become a doctor.

To my dad, who always told me, "Once a job has begun, never leave it till it is done. Be that labor great or small, do it well or not at all." I am much fonder of that statement now that I am grown. I also would never be so versed in show tunes if I didn't hear him singing and humming them in the early morning before I was fully awake.

To my mom, I don't know how to even start. You are the single most influential person in my life and I am grateful for you. You are truly the greatest mom ever. It is a fact; even other people tell me this. Your love and caring is never ending. You have always been there to guide me and give me advice and still love me, even if I didn't take it. Words fall short of what you mean to me, and all that I can say is thank you for being you. There is no one else like you in the world.

To my love, you have grown right before my eyes and became more than I ever could have imagined you to be. You are a wonderful person and soul. Thank you for being there. You make everything better.

I think that is it. I hope I have and will continue to add to everyone's life. I love you all. Thank you for being on this journey with me. We have seen what the past has gifted us with, and I look forward to all the future has to offer. Have faith in the universe and it will be our keeper.

Table of Contents

Foreword:
Why I Wrote This Book

Life is a journey. Like yours, my life has taken many twists and turns as I've learned new things about myself and the power of healing.

Entering college as an exercise physiology major some years ago, I thought that if I just learned about ailments of the body and how to manage them, I could help people wracked by pain and ill health. But something was missing. Yes, I knew that getting and keeping people in good physical shape was important, but many were still sick.

So I turned to a new form of study and healing: chiropractic care. I was certain that by learning how to heal my patients from the inside out, I would be more successful. I was wrong. A piece was still missing for some patients, a very important piece: the mind and body connection to healing.

It has taken me years to figure out how this connection works in the way people heal. The information that I've gathered, and the experiences that I've had have thrust me forward on a new quest, one that sets me on a course to treat people in a whole new way by helping them find the mind and body connection necessary for good health and a happier, more fulfilled life. And now I want to share it with you!

The mind and body connection is powerful. I know; I've experienced it. After working for years in the field of exercise physiology and as a doctor of chiropractic, I've learned an important lesson: true healing comes from within. Yes, you *can* use your mind to help heal yourself. Or you can use it to sabotage any attempt of physical, emotional, or spiritual progress. Unfortunately, far too many people don't use their own inner power to help themselves. Why? Because they don't know how.

Everyone has action potential—those things within us that can help us become better, stronger, and healthier people. Within the pages of this book, I will help you to discover *Your Action Potential,* in order to enable you to make better decisions about your own health and express a true, innate life force.

I've designed this book as a roadmap on a new journey: one that will lead you through a process that gives you all of the information you need to realign your life so that it can work for *you,* and not *against you.*

We cannot live in a *"should"* type of world. Instead, we need to create a world where it is our obligation (to ourselves and to our loved ones), to get the best information we can and pass it on to everyone we know.

That's what this book is all about—passing on what I've learned through years of study in order to help you get the results you want and need from your life.

Within these pages, my goal is to ignite your interest and challenge all that you think you already know as true by looking at yourself and your world from a whole new angle in order to see it more clearly.

If there's one thing that I want to impart on you, dear reader, it's the importance of *you*! For years I tried to treat ailing people with either physical exercise therapy or chiropractic care, only to realize that some people are their own worst enemies. They couldn't get better no matter what therapy we tried because they hadn't yet learned how to help themselves on their personal journey toward recovery. Their road was blocked. If yours is too, isn't it time you took a detour? If you find yourself not getting the results you want in either your health or your life situation, or you find yourself working way too hard for the results you are getting, it may be time to step headlong into this journey with me—one that will test you in a way you've never been tested before by taking you step-by-step through the process of learning to give yourself the support you both need and deserve! Sound easy? Well, it won't be! Learning to become your own number one cheerleader isn't natural for most of us and must be practiced. But it can be done, and trust me when I say the results are spectacular!

Health happens from the inside out. It takes awareness and a commitment to work with your body to heal your body. But you can do it with the right tools, of course!

Now it is time to start your journey with me. Let's take a closer look at *Your Action Potential.*

What Does Action Potential Have to Do with Me?

Everything you want in life—a great job, a healthier body, a more loving relationship, even more money—is right there, ready for you to take hold of! So what's stopping you? The odds are it's *Your Action Potential*—or lack of it.

So, what is this buzzword we keep throwing out here: *Your Action Potential?* I'm glad you asked. Let's look at it from its most basic component: the life of a single cell.

Action Potential happens within the cells of the body when it is "charged" beyond its threshold. The threshold is the relation of an electrical charge inside of the cell versus the charge on the outside of the cell. *Action Potential* gives your entire body the energy (some may call it the motivation) it needs to move forward.

When a cell is charged from the inside, it reaches a

threshold which, although there is energy, nothing is "happening." Now, add just a tiny bit of external energy, and *pow*! An enormous gain in energy is released.

So, how does this relate to *Your Action Potential*? It is the release of this external energy that enables you to plow forward in life in order to attain your optimal health and happiness.

It's sad to see how many people are walking around having never attained their lifelong dreams. I hope to change that! Everyone I have ever worked with has been so close to a solution to their physical, medical, and emotional problems and just couldn't see it for themselves. So, what's the problem?

One main obstacle I have noticed is the broken spirit. While one person may face a challenge and over-come it to achieve great success, another may find it too difficult and allow their spirit to be broken, which also causes a break in energy. The longer someone remains in this state of brokenness, the longer it takes—and the more energy it requires—to find their way back to their optimal state of well-being.

You know how it works. You've seen it happen. Or maybe you've lived it. Something unexpected strikes: an illness, a layoff, a divorce, or worse. One person sees it as a challenge and overcomes with striking results. Another simply wallows in their misfortune, failing to fight, and ultimately getting sicker, more miserable, and far worse off than when they started.

Or maybe you've simply let life take over. So many of us get into jobs, relationships, and "situations" that literally sap our energy, taking so much of our time and energy that we simply can't move forward and are stuck running on a treadmill to nowhere.

This is no way to live, and you know it. Now's the time to break these destructive cycles and find *Your Action Potential* in order to live the life you were destined for. How? You do this by adding a little "laser-focused stimulus" to your life (and your cells) in order to get moving. *Your Action Potential* is closer than you think. Now, let's find it!

Becoming a Super Ball and Not Super Glue

"Where are you in life, and where do you want to go?" Sounds like a simple enough question, now doesn't it? Think hard and be honest. It may not be as easy as you first thought. I am always surprised at how many people I work with have no idea where they are in life and where they're headed. They just seem to keep plugging forward with little or no thought.

It's time to start investigating your life journey. Think of life as a road trip. Now, if you were headed to places unknown, where would you begin? Chances are, you'd get out a map and find your starting place and your ending destination and chart the easiest route to get there.

From this plan, you would gather additional information to make your journey easier, which may include:

- an estimate of the miles to be traveled
- a timeframe for the trip
- a calculation of travel costs
- accommodations available
- a list of food items to take to eliminate stops

Now, this list could go on and on depending on how in-depth and organized you are. The more information you can gather about the roads, rest areas, and accommodations you'll encounter, the easier your trip ought to be. Decide to simply jump in the car with little thought or planning and you're bound to encounter difficulties along the way.

Think about the way you would plan a big trip. Now, take those same concepts and incorporate them into your daily decision-making. Think about all of the time, emotion, and money that you could save if you just looked at the "whole picture" every time you needed to make a decision, both large and small. Sound simplistic? Well, it is. But that doesn't mean that it doesn't work!

Now, let's take this simple system and throw in a big wrench—we'll call it *life*. Yes, life does have a way of throwing obstacles in our path and making us change direction mid-trip. But there is a way to get to your goals more quickly and allow you to turn more of your dreams into reality than you ever thought possible. It's the power of the super ball.

Yes, I said "super ball." You know, that little, bouncing ball that seem to zip across the room, gaining momentum and speed as they whiz by? Now, think about the types of people you know. Chances are some are like those super balls (always whizzing by, getting things done), and some are like Super glue (always stuck in the same spot, never moving forward by much, unable to go after their dreams).

Now, don't get me wrong, Super glue is great for sticking things together, but when you let that analogy run your life, you're bound to get stuck in a sort of limbo.

Compare that to the super ball personalities, who like their namesake gain momentum when they encounter an obstacle and speed up in response to anything negative and escape its outcome. The super ball personality has the tendency to "go for it" no matter what the challenge. This can be a great motivator in chasing your dreams and attaining health and unity in your life.

Think about it. The go-getters out there who always manage to get things done are all super balls. They may not always have "a path," but they always manage to persevere.

Here comes the big question: are you a super ball? If not, why? After all, it's the super balls who are successful.

Maybe you aren't really sure, or you want to be a super ball and just don't know where to start. Here are ten main traits that set super balls apart from everyone else—especially *super glues*:

1.   **Spiritually Healthy.** Usually calm and centered, these people are always grounded in the face of adversity.

2.   **Balance-centered.** Striving for a balance of mind, body, relationship, and wealth, these individuals believe in the connection between health and balance.

3.   **Visionary.** Most able to see what they want in their mind, with true vision, they are able to envision an end result and devise a plan to get there.

4.   **Priority-managed.** Super balls tend to tackle the worst things first, allowing them to do the things they like least early so they can enjoy more relaxing and enjoyable activities as the day wears on.

5.   **Planner.** Once a vision is considered, the planner creates steps toward achieving it.

6.   **Organizer.** Super balls understand business systems and division of labor. Everything is done the same way every time in order to avoid unnecessary mistakes. They also strive to give everyone jobs that best fit their talents and interest.

7.   **Leaders.** These folks have the ability to understand and execute influence and negotiation in all situations.

8.   **Good Presenters.** The ability to communicate thoughts and ideas in such a fashion so large, diverse groups actually "get it."

9. **Financially Savvy.** Super balls are smart with money. They know how to make it; use it, and invest it.

10. **Asset Protection and Tax-planning.** Knowing how to protect your money and plan for the future is an important trait for taking good care of yourself and taking full advantage of your assets.

Look at these traits. Be honest with yourself. Do any of them fit your personality, or do you have some work to do to become a true super ball? Next, I'm going to show you how to improve your super ball skills in three easy steps. This system is called psycho-neuro duplication. Ready? Now try this:

Step #1: Say the words "I am ____." This could be "I am the greatest presenter in the world," or "I am the greatest doctor. Everyone I treat gets exceptional outcomes." This isn't something you necessarily need to believe about yourself right now, but something you'd like to be true about you.

Step #2: Gather all the data you can on how a person with these characteristics would act.

Step #3: Act as if it is already true. Fake it until you make it true in a good way. Remember, reality is created by validation.

Now, does this simple system seem difficult or out of reach? I would say not. Yet, think of the implications using such a system can have on your life. Let me give you an example:

1. "I am a healthy and amazing public speaker."

2. Gather all of the available data about how an amazing speaker would act. One good way to do this is to find an already successful public speaker that you enjoy and copy his/her attributes. Or look up a few well-known speakers online, read their books, watch their videos, and attend one of their seminars. Study their mannerisms, their speech patterns, even their tone. Research their background. If at all possible, set up a meeting or paid consultation with them.

Take a risk and ask them how to accomplish this yourself. You may be surprised at how responsive some people can be when the situation is handled correctly. Say something like, "I have done some research on you and would like to take you to a restaurant of your choice and treat you to dinner while we talk about how you have become such an amazing speaker."

I know this may sound like strange request, but if you truly feel this way about a person, it would be hard for them to say no to such a heartfelt and honest request.

In the event the person you most want to speak with denies your request, don't stop there. Be a super ball and move on to the next person on your list. There's a lot to be learned. You just have to find someone willing to open up and share their insight.

3. Act as if what you've said about yourself is already true. Now is the time to show off your stuff. Don't be shy. Using the speaking example once again; start applying what you have learned. Test it out. Begin speaking on topics that you are most knowledgeable and comfortable with anywhere you can: at work, your children's school, church, even at the local community center. Find opportunities to practice your new skills. That's the only way to improve.

These are the traits necessary to become everything you were ever meant to be and more than you ever thought you could become. Using the top ten traits of super balls, you will be able to truly evaluate yourself. With this list, you will be able to know which traits you have, and hone in on the ones that you need a little help with.

Welcome to the super balls of the world! Look toward others with these traits, and you will see yourself improving day by day as you journey toward the healthy, fulfilled person you've always dreamed you could be.

Discovering What
Happiness Means to You

If there's a secret to true happiness, it may be this: happiness means different things to different people. Accept that. What makes your neighbor, your sister, or even your spouse happy may have little or no impact whatsoever on the way you feel. Now, that may sound obvious, but the truth is that far too many of us seek out things that seem to make *other* people happy in a quest to feel better with very little regard to what makes *us* happy.

The simple fact is people get unhappy when they don't get the thing or outcome they think they want. They want a new house, and when they can't get a mortgage they can afford, they're unhappy. Or maybe they want their spouse to be more affectionate, and when they aren't, they decide their marriage is in shambles. With so much emphasis on outward things to make us happy, it's no wonder so many people today rely on medications to feel good.

Considering what makes us unhappy, wouldn't it make more sense to simply readjust your wants whenever feelings of unhappiness arise? Yet, few of us are able to "let go" of our expectations—even when it means finding the contentment and happiness in our lives that we crave.

Let's look at some people who are happy. You know the type, the man or women, that no matter what life throws their way finds a silver lining? Annoying, aren't they? Yet, they have a lot to teach us. Many may wonder if such people are truly happy or just faking it.

Research has proven that most happy people share a few common characteristics—and you might be surprised at what they are.

Most of us tend to think that "things" bring happiness. They don't. Just look at your friends, co-workers, neighbors, and family members with the most money, best car, nicest-looking kids, and interesting job. Are they really the happiest people you know? Take a close look. According to recent research, those superficial factors may make life *easier*, but it doesn't necessarily make you h*appier*.

Consider this interesting fact: it has been shown that a strong, positive relationship between your job status, income, wealth, and happiness only exists for those who live below the poverty line and/or who are unemployed. Amazing! Does that mean you have to be down on your luck to really be happy? Absolutely not!

It does mean, however, that you don't need things

(or even security) to be happy. What distinguishes happy people from the rest of us is their attitude. They are usually the freethinkers who go their own way and don't always try to please everyone else or keep up with what society believes you should do, have, or even the way you should act.

Look around at the truly happy people in your life. The odds are they live *differently*. Maybe very differently than what you would call "normal." That's why they're happy! They aren't running around like crazy trying to fit in or be something they aren't. They know who they are, what they like (and want), and what they don't—and they're content with that!

I remember a gentleman I met years ago. He had a great job, and it was obvious he had some money. Yet, this man always drove a rickety old car, wore off-the-rack clothes (even though he could afford tailor-made suits), and settled for camping with his family in lieu of expensive whirlwind vacations. I asked him once why he didn't enjoy his money more.

His answer was surprising. "I do," he said. "I just choose to enjoy the money I have right now in my pocket and not the money I think I have in investments or on my credit cards or in the equity of my house. I intentionally live below my means so that I can enjoy life without stress and worry about paying the bills. I don't need a new car. I do need to take time off to attend each and every one of my son's baseball games. Being debt-free gives me the freedom to do just that. I am not obligated to work overtime because I don't need to.

I have never forgotten that conversation. In the three minutes we spoke, I learned a lifetime of lessons from that gentleman.

Today that man is fifty-two years old and is retired and living out the rest of his days (which will be numerous) doing what he wants when he wants and truly enjoying his life. Now, that would make anyone happy!

Why Is Being Happy Important?

It may seem obvious; after all, who wants to be unhappy? But the implications of being happy may be far greater than you might think. The fact is that happier people are also healthier people—something we all strive for. So how do we attain true happiness?

American psychologist Martin Seligan is known for his "equation for happiness":

H = S + C + V

H = Happiness
S = Set range (genetics: about 50%)
C = Circumstances (8–15%)
V = Voluntary Control (past, present, future)

This may be difficult to understand at first, but is really quite simple:

Set Range/Genetics - It is believed we are each born with a certain amount of "set happiness" that is determined by our genes and contributes to about half of our level of happiness. Regardless of what we do, this set happiness isn't supposed to be able to change much.

Circumstances - While many people believe that their life circumstances play a huge role in their level of happiness, it really is quite low according to statistics— only about eight to fifteen percent. That's good news for those who haven't had the "happiest" of lives up until now.

Voluntary Control - This may be the most important factor that helps determine your personal happiness, especially since you control it. Voluntary control includes the way you think, act, and react to the things and people in your life and accounts for almost forty-two percent of your happiness ratio.

Your Past - There's no use dwelling on the bad stuff that has happened in the past, and happy people know it! Those who experience true happiness tend to focus on happier times and feelings and let the rest go. The simple fact is, the way you think and act right now is essential in determining how happy you are today and will be in the future.

Yes, You Do Have Control over Your Happiness

It's easy to see from this equation that you do have some control over your happiness even though some factors are indeed out of your control. You can choose to control your attitude, the way you interpret situations, and even the way you think about yourself (we'll discuss this in more detail in later chapters). If you think about it, you control nearly fifty percent of your happiness at any given moment! Isn't it time you took control of your happiness and changed the way you feel from minute to minute, hour to hour, and day to day?

So, does that mean you can't ever be sad? Of course not! In fact, those who've experienced rough patches in life often report enjoying the good, joyous times even more. Sadness is a part of life. Don't deny it. It offers its own lessons.

As we've learned, happiness is something that means different things to different people, but basically, what makes each of us happy is the way we think about ourselves, our place in the world and the world around us, plus the way we act in that world. So in order to find true happiness, you first need to discover what makes *you* happy.

Sidebar:

20 *Things to Make You Happy*
You choose to be happy or miserable. So why not find a few things to smile about right now? Here's a list to get you started:

1.   The fact that you are alive (Even if you aren't feeling your best today, you're still here.)

2.   A warm bubble bath waiting for you tonight

3.   The people who put up with you (and love you despite yourself)

4.   The opportunity to choose what direction your life will lead

5.   Warm, toasty socks in the middle of winter

6. Your favorite meal—or dessert!

7. Hobbies that help us enjoy life!

8. Exercise—yes, even exercise can help brighten your mood!

9. A light rain shower

10. Rainbows

11. An unexpected letter or phone call from an old friend

12. The five dollar bill you found tucked in your jacket pocket

13. Sales at your favorite store!

14. Your IRS refund

15. Vacations

16. Warm, sunny days

17. Sultry summer nights

18. Sexy negligees for yourself or someone special

19. A good book

20. A great joke

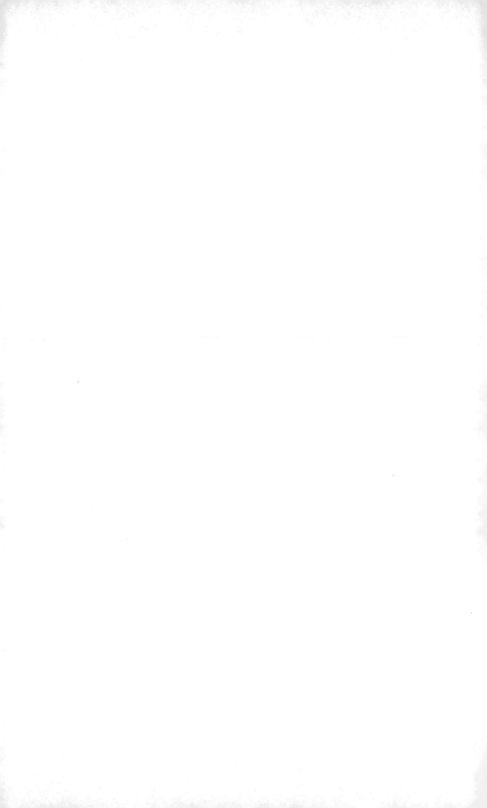

The Secrets of Success

Success Defined

Success, like happiness, is a personal thing. Everyone rates success differently—as well, they should. Understanding this is the first step to achieving the success that you're after.

So, what is success? Basically, it is "the completion of anything intended." In other words, success is finishing what you planned to do. Whew! And so many of us have been stuck thinking that success only meant making the most money, having the most high-powered job, or driving a $100,000 car!

On the contrary, a truly successful person sets out to do something (anything), and then does just that! Simply put, make a plan—any plan—and follow it, and you have succeeded! Sounds simple enough, doesn't it? Then why do only eighty-five percent of us actually finish what we start? The reason may be our inability to take charge of the situations we face instead of simply reacting to them.

There are two basic ways of dealing with any situation: we can either act or react to it. When we react, we base our actions and emotions on everything else. We are allowing everything around us to actually gauge our response to what's happening. Sounds a bit tiring, doesn't it? It is, and chances are that's the way you have been handling the situations in your life for years. Simply taking a moment to act instead of react will free up a tremendous amount of energy for you to use to find your life potential as the energy you save in these situations is invested into higher efforts that lead to success.

Your Success—Your Choice

When it comes to success, you be the judge. No one can, or should, tell you what makes you a success or a failure. It's completely up to you! Now, isn't that a liberating thought? Well, it's true.

The first step to attaining personal success is a simple one: determining what it is. We've already discussed the definition of success: completing what you set out to do. The question is what do you want to do? You need to know what your idea of success is before you can move forward. But how do you do that? I have a few exercises for you to try to get to the core of your this issue.

The first thing I want you to do is take out a clean sheet of paper (you may need several) and one of your favorite pens. Write the word success at the top of the first page. Now, look at the word. Start writing. No stopping now. Keep writing. Jot down everything that comes to mind when you think of the word success. Do this for ten minutes uninterrupted. No cheating now. No stopping. No thinking. Just writing.

Some of you may find this exercise a bit difficult, because you've never really thought about what success means to you. Others will have no trouble filling a page or more with thoughts, quips, words, and more. Be careful not to filter any of your answers. We'll evaluate them later.

Okay, time's up. Now let's check out that list. Are you surprised by what you wrote? Don't be. This is what you really think of success. Now, take another sheet of paper and begin to rewrite your list by order of importance with the most important being on the top, of course. If there are things you aren't sure about, either refine them a bit to better fit your list or throw them out. It's up to you.

Once complete, you'll have your own personal list of what makes you feel successful. Keep it; you'll need it in the future. After all, you can't hit a target if you don't know where (or what) the target is.

Moving Forward: Attaining Your Dreams in Five Years

Now that you have a personal definition for success in front of you, it's time to put it into action. I have wonderful news for you: you can have virtually everything you want in the next five years! Never thought it possible, did you? Well, it is! This is where the fun begins.

Now, maybe you're thinking that attaining true success takes longer than five years. I ask you, why? Let's face it. We're each only here for a set number of years, and we don't have time to waste. It's time to shake things up and get moving. Success is only an arms length away. Isn't it time you grabbed hold of it?

It's time to set your targets so that you can hit them. Now, let's get started. But first, let me give you one suggestion: always reach higher than you thought you could. Your power to create anything in your life is limitless, so don't limit yourself now.

Now, we're going to develop your Dream Sheet. Grab a new sheet of paper, and let's get working. Begin by asking yourself what you want to achieve in the next five years with the thought that everything you write on this sheet *will* happen in the next five years. Include people you want to meet, places you want to go, things you want to do, awards you want to receive—anything and everything!

This is a pretty cool drill, but it gets cooler. The fact that you are actually writing down your dreams gives it greater potential for coming true. The simple action of writing gets the concepts into your conscious and subconscious mind to make them a reality in your life.

Okay, now here goes. Begin writing for five minutes. Write down everything you want in the next five years. If it doesn't make it to the sheet, it won't happen. You must give this exercise your total and undivided attention. Without it, it can't be effective. Ready, set, go!

Finished? Good. Now take list number one and list number two and compare them. Notice anything? List number two is the things that you are truly able to achieve without all of those negative, subconscious controls you may have put on your first list.

Hard to believe that all of these things are right at your fingertips, isn't it? Well, don't be surprised. They are! As soon as you let yourself believe that attaining all of these wonders is possible, it is!

Take this dream sheet and keep it somewhere where you can look at it every day. There has been research to back up the fact that writing down your dreams and reviewing them on a regular basis helps them indeed come true.

Now, just one more exercise. This one is designed to give you clarity. Clarity is an incredible thing. You have no chance of hitting your target if you have no idea what to aim at. Clarity helps to bring your target into focus.

Now, I'm going to ask you a question, and I need the first thing that pops into your head. Okay, here goes. Describe your perfect day at work. What about a perfect day at play? Sit down and describe these two days.

Finally, close your eyes and picture the person you know that wouldn't be happy even if you gave them a million dollars. You know there's someone in your life like that.

Once you've completed these exercises, you'll have a much better idea when you hit your target and what to do to aim better when you miss. By making these commitments to yourself, you are finding clarity. Notice how it feels. Pretty good, doesn't it? Now that you have focus and aim, your perfect days and dreams are finally within reach. Grab them!

Sidebar:

Tips for Success
There are a lot of ways to feel successful that have little (or nothing) to do with money. Just because you don't have a high-powered job on Wall Street, or live in a nine hundred square foot house vs. a nine thousand square foot one doesn't mean that you're a failure. If you are content with what you have and what you are doing, then I'd say you are more successful than those who have a lot more "things" and a lot less contentment.

But what if you want more? Here are a few tips to finding the success you're after:

Figure out what you really want (not what you think you should have to fit in). For instance, do you really want to be a doctor, or would the schedule of a nurse better fit the other things you want out of life?

- Don't be intimidated—either by other's expectations or your own. Don't let anyone dictate what you should do. Be happy with your own level of success. After all, you have to live with it! On the flip side, don't be afraid to go after a dream—even if it seems beyond your reach. If you really want it, it's yours for the taking!

- Devise a plan and stick to it. Ask anyone who's gone after their dreams and reached them how in the world they did it, and they'll all say they had a plan. You know what you want, now figure out the best route to getting it!

Sidebar:

What Does Success Really Mean?
Want to learn more about success and what it really means? Check out some of these quotes:

"Try not to be a man of success, but rather to be a man of value."

—Albert Einstein

"Unless a man undertakes more than he possibly can do, he will never do all that he can."

—Henry Drummond

"Footprints on the sands of time are not made by sitting down."

—unknown

"Greatness lies not in being strong, but in the right use of strength."

—Henry Ward Beecher

"Nothing will ever be attempted if all possible objections must first be overcome."

—Samuel Johnson

"Do what you can, with what you have, where you are."

—Theodore Roosevelt

"The world can only be grasped by action, not by contemplation... The hand is the cutting edge of the mind."

—Jacob Bronowski

"It is time for us to stand and cheer for the doer, the achiever, the one who recognizes the challenge and does something about it."

—Vince Lombardi

"Many of life's failures are people who did not realize how close they were to success when they gave up."

—Thomas Edison

"What would you attempt to do if you knew you would not fail?"

—Robert Schuller

"We never know how far reaching something we may think, say, or do today will affect the lives of millions tomorrow."

—B.J. Palmer

"The tragedy in life doesn't lie in not reaching your goal. The tragedy lies in having no goal to reach."

—Benjamin Mays

Being Your Own Cheerleader!

You can be your greatest ally or your biggest enemy. Most people never realize they are the one stopping them from getting everything they want out of life. Scary thought, isn't it? To think, you really are responsible for what happens to you!

There's an old saying that goes, "There are a million excuses and never a good reason." The time for excuses is over. Today, you begin owning your own life. Instead of letting life happen to you, you're now going to make life happen! Once you begin to do this, you can take all of that energy you've been expending on things that don't really matter and put it toward higher return activities. You know the ones that really count!

Now that you have taken ultimate responsibility for your life, you have to make sure that you're really on board. *Well, of course I am*, you think. *Why else would I be reading this book?*

True, but I know from the experience of coaching and training many people that far too many think they're on board for change, yet as soon as they get close to attaining their dreams, they allow "something" to go wrong. That "something" is usually themselves.

"How can anyone be their own worst enemy?" you may ask. It happens all of the time! The reason usually has to do with a complex psychological theory called subconscious programming.

So, what is subconscious programming? Essentially, it is a database that we are not consciously aware of that is built within us by all of the things that were said to us in our early years. These could have been statements made by others, or even ones made to ourselves about ourselves. Consider this: as soon as someone lets words roll off their tongue, they are embedded in us—stuck in this database—until we purposefully kick them out. The trouble is few of us even know that they're there.

Now, these words can be good words, or they can be bad words. For instance, if you did not get the raise you think you deserved, you can either give yourself good words like, "I know I deserved it; there must be some other reason why my boss denied my request," or you could use bad, destructive words like, "I'm so stupid; I couldn't even get a raise!" Now, your body takes those words and begins to believe them. Your mind and body will unconsciously use those words to thwart any attempt at success—if you allow it to. So, the next time you are about to berate yourself, remember this: you are in control of what you input into your database. This simple thought may help you tame your words and give yourself the good words you need to succeed more often.

Now, sometimes we have no control over the words put into our database. Take, for instance, the child who is constantly berated and scorned. Their database is being filled with destructive words that can hinder their ability to succeed later in life. Meanwhile, the child who has positive reinforcement may do better in school, have more friends, and even seem happier. Is child number two better, stronger, or smarter than child number one? Probably not. Their database is just filled with more good things than bad. Without more positive data, they may not internally feel worthy of success and goodness and actually spend their lives sabotaging their own efforts at success.

Most people with low self-esteem have very high negative data and low positive data in their base. However, most of us fall somewhere in the middle with a little of both.

In order to reach your true *Action Potential*, you must be willing to take charge of what you allow to stay in your subconscious database, and get rid of the rest. What you appear like to yourself will ultimately be how you appear to the outside world.

When and only when, you begin to feel that all good things should be happening to you, not because the world owes it to you, but because you deserve it, then those good things will begin to happen. It's the law of the universe. Give good things to it, and it will give good things to you.

I feel it necessary at this point to clarify the fact that you should be using the energy of the universe to power you in all you do, even your daily tasks. After all, the universe has an endless supply of energy, so why not use it? Chinese medicine relies heavily on this concept using ch'i (which can be recharged and used in conjunction with the universe) and your own personal jing, or life force.

It is believed that once your jing is gone, your life is over. There's nothing you can do to replace it. So, what's the solution? The Chinese believe it is to never use it, relying solely on the ch'i.

Of course, it is important to recharge the ch'i, lest you risk tapping into that all-important jing. To do this, you must get sufficient sleep, nutrition, water, and relaxation.

Now, when you grow tired and need a rest, ask the universe for help with your energy level. Doubting that this will work? Try it. Imagine how powerful it would be to get tired and run out of energy only when you are ready to rest and not before.

Still doubtful? Think of it is this way: look at yourself as an electrical conductor that regularly takes energy from the universe. You have the ability to run energy through you and harness it to get everything done in your life that needs to be done and more. The universe is alive and pulsing with energy that is readily available to suit all of your needs. All you need to do is learn to harness it. Then and only then will you have the ability to be as productive as you want with little need for rest. This is the prescription for *success*.

Ever wonder how the most successful people you know never seem to run out of energy, going non-stop from morning until late into the evening? This is how they do it!

Setting Your Path with One Simple Exercise

Now, let's talk about the finger-pointing exercise. "What is it?" you ask. Well, I'm going to tell you. This is a simple exercise designed to help you keep yourself aligned, with an eye toward your goals. Chances are you have a good idea when you're working against yourself in a situation. Now we're going to take that knowledge and put it to work in your favor.

The best way to achieve your goals is to work toward them, right? Yet, many of us still manage to thwart our own efforts. Why? Because we find it hard to believe that *everything we do counts*, and it either works for us or against us. So every time you have a decision to make, ask yourself, "Is this going to help me get closer to my goals?" If the answer that comes to mind right away is no, then don't waste your time or energy. Remember, the first answer that pops into your head is usually the true answer. You may feel compelled to justify your answer or even change it—don't! Resisting the truth will only delay your progress and strip you of your ability to achieve your goals.

Breaking Bad Habits

Good habits are as easy to build up as bad ones, so go for the things that have a greater good. But, let's face it; breaking bad habits isn't always an easy task. That's where the finger-pointing exercise comes in handy. Whenever you are going to do something that is going to move you away from your goals, take your pointer finger on the hand you use the most, and point it right at your face. Now, you may not want to do this in front of people, lest they think you a bit crazy. This is a great way to set yourself straight (which really means telling yourself the truth) and remind yourself what you need to do to be successful. No longer will you hinder your own personal development. With this exercise, you are forced to face the truth and make a decision either for or against yourself. The choice is yours. Just remember, you have to live with the consequences.

Use this technique often and with consistency, and it will serve you well. Everything you do from now on will express a true transformation toward the life you crave.

Everyone already knows the answers to the questions in their lives. Sometimes you just need a little help to realize your own personal *Action Potential*. Each and every exercise I give you in this book has been designed to have a synergistic effect with the next one you use. What this means is that you have a great return on your investment. One plus one now equals ten. I love when this happens in my life … and you will too!

Sidebar:

Are You Your Own Worst Enemy? Take This Quiz and Find Out!

Far too many of us thwart our own efforts toward success. Without even realizing it, we sabotage any effort at accomplishing our goals and getting the life we want and deserve. Are you your own worst enemy? Answer yes or no to the following questions:

1. Do I often bad-talk to myself, telling myself I'm stupid, ugly, fat, and worthless, or anything else that's negative?

2. Do I often get close to achieving a goal, only to have "something" happen at the last minute to stop it from happening?

3. Do I often put off going after my dreams?

4. Am I often too exhausted to even try something new?

5. Do I often feel unworthy—like someone else deserves things more than I do?

If you answered yes to one or more of these questions, you could possibly be sabotaging your own efforts. Take the time now to learn how to speak kindly to yourself, gather energy from the universe, and accept the fact that yes, you are worth it! Your dreams are yours for the taking. Isn't it time that you grabbed for them?

Simple Steps to Achieving Your Dreams

Don't be afraid to think big—or even small! Once you know what you want, the rest is relatively easy. Just follow the simple steps below to touch the stars.

- **Find a Passion**. Wanting something a little bit isn't enough—you have to want it a lot! It is said that the starting point of achievement is desire. To reach your goals, you must truly feel passionate about the dream you set forth. Otherwise, it simply won't be worth the work. So look inside of yourself and discover where your passion lies. Now. You're ready to go get it!

- **Visualize yourself reaching your goal**. The truth is you are the commander of your own ship. If you want something badly enough and are willing to work hard enough to get it, you will. Nothing can stop a machine in motion—especially one passionate about their goals. Let yourself see and feel what achieving your dreams will be like. Ask yourself how it will change the things and people around you—especially you! Visualize success, and it will come! If you find it difficult to visualize yourself achieving your goals, chances are you won't.

- **Plan for It!** Achieving success doesn't come easily. It requires a thorough and thought-out plan. Remember the road trip we talked about earlier? Well, it's time to set your course. Create simple action steps to get you started. Follow them consistently every day, and soon you'll notice that you are indeed on your way.

- **Make a commitment.** You've already written down your dreams in the previous chapter. Now keep it posted somewhere where it can be easily seen. Make a commitment to work toward it on a regular basis. Set a timeline for success. This will give you the needed push to get moving and keep moving toward your goals.

- **Review your progress on a regular basis.** Make sure you are making—and continue to make—progress. Don't let your dreams just fade away. Take action!

Of course, there's still more work for us to do, but keep all of these tips in mind as we move forward toward the life you're dreaming of.

Victors, Not Victims!

If you want to be successful, there's one simple truth you must come to grips with: it's impossible to be successful and productive when you are a victim! Never!

Sure, everyone has had things happen to them in the past, but you simply cannot let those things rule your today, your present, if you want to reach for the stars. That doesn't in any way imply that I do not feel compassion for those who have survived horrible things happening to them. It's just important to understand how destructive remaining a victim can be to your life. Victims are controlled and overwhelmed by their past. They are frozen in it, unable to move forward. Not a pleasant place to be, to say the least.

Let me make this more real for you. Think about a person in your life. You know the one that no one else wants to ask, "How is your day?" for fear of the answer. Everyone knows someone like this. They are the perpetual victim who always has "something" going wrong in their life: their car is broken, their kids are sick, their mother-in-law just moved in.

Have this person in your mind right now? Now, how does it feel to be around this person? Is it warm and motivating or exhausting, giving you the feeling that you want and need to escape their clutches? Chances are you can't get away fast enough. Is this the person that *you* want to be? I thought not. And, if you are, don't worry, change is in the air.

To be a victor, you must be able to take misfortune and learn from it. Nothing is totally bad—really. Every challenge offers a lesson and an opportunity to make something good come from it; maybe not today, maybe not tomorrow, but someday in the future. This process turns the most downcast person into someone who is able to "spin" everything that happens to them into a web of greatness—or at least goodness.

Life is full of challenges. No, not problems. I said challenges. These challenges are designed to make you stronger. Before you know it, they'll turn you into a decision-making machine! This will save you many things, the greatest being time.

Now, let's take a closer look at time. Consider this: time is one of the only things in life that you can't get back. Once it's gone, it's gone forever. You can earn back money. You buy back a car, a house, sometimes even a lost spouse. But you can never, ever replace time.

I have a real eye-opener for you. Let's take a look at the life equation of time. Are you ready? Here it is: take your age and subtract it from how old you think you'll live to be, then subtract another five years. Now you are looking at your true life in years. Shocking, isn't it?

We've all heard the old adage: "It isn't the years in your life but the life in your years." Few things in life are truer. Ask yourself, does it really matter if you live to a hundred and fifty if all of those years are filled with pain and suffering? I certainly hope not!

Maybe you're already midway through your life. The sad fact is that if you continue to do things the same old way tomorrow that you did today and last week and last month, then you will continue to yield the same results. Now, if you're happy with those results, so be it. Good for you. But the fact that you are reading this book tells a different story.

Some say that the definition of insanity is *doing the same thing over and over and expecting a different result.* If that's you, then I'm sorry to say the world considers you insane—a sobering thought, to say the least. Luckily, you have help—me! Now is your chance to make a change and get off the treadmill to nowhere that you have been running on.

A huge step toward knowing what you want is knowing what you do *not* want. You do not want to be insane, so changes must be made.

Future back thinking is a great place to start. This technique requires having a goal in mind, then working backward toward that goal. Here's an example: you want to buy a house. What do you need to do to make this purchase happen? First, you need a down payment, plus a credit score that's high enough to get you a loan approval at a good rate on a mortgage.

Let's say that you would like your down payment to equal at least $100,000—a lofty goal, to be sure. That would mean that you would have to bank $20,000 a year for the next five years (our deadline for attaining your dreams, remember?). The more precise you can make your goal, the better chance you will have of turning it into a reality.

Here's way to take this scenario even further. Twenty-thousand dollars over five years (260 weeks), equals $77 per week—a bit less daunting a figure to work with. Now, with this in mind, it may not seem out of the realm of possibility to save $150 a week and decrease your savings time from five years to just two and a half years. Wow! This method allows you to set goals based on facts, not a shot in the dark. It's a method that can be applied to any goal. The trick is to continue to break it down until it is in a more manageable state. That will enable you to better handle the challenge set forth and set your victim days behind you in lieu of a place in line with your fellow victors in the land of victory!

Passion: The Key to Success

Choose something you love, and make oodles of cash doing it. Sounds simple enough, but is it practical? "Yes!" say the experts. As a matter of fact, it's the only way to attain the kind of success most of us only dream about.

When President George W. Bush called Baby Einstein creator and founder, Julie Aigner-Clark, one of America's "most talented business entrepreneurs," during his 2007 State of the Union address, you could hear moms across America cheering. Why? After all, she was one of them. The only difference between the well-groomed businesswoman being hailed by the president and those watching from behind a burp cloth was the fact that she was the one with the guts to take her passion and run all the way to the bank with it.

Julie Aigner-Clark knows what all successful people know (both men and women): passion equals success! And boy does she know all about success. In 2001, she sold her fledging little company to the Disney company for an undisclosed amount of money. At the time, Baby Einstein was estimated to be worth more than $10 million! Not bad for an $18,000 initial investment a few years earlier!

So, how did this average, everyday mom go from new mommy to mommy millionaire, virtually overnight? She created a dream, devised a plan, and saw it through to reality. Of course, she never intended on her baby videos becoming a household name. All she really wanted was to create something that she thought would interest her own young daughter. See how our dreams have the tendency to grow bigger than we ever imagined if only we get out of their way?

Living by the number one rule of "making it big," Julie took her passion for classical music, science, and poetry, and coupling it with her interest in exposing her young toddler to these arts, created a product that helped fill a void and made what is admittedly the most influential infant development media product of our time.

Maybe you aren't interested in becoming a multi-millionaire. That's okay. Being successful doesn't mean making lots of money or attending dinner at the White House. It does mean discovering what will make you happy in life and doing whatever you have to make it happen. You can't do that if you dread getting up every morning and heading out the door to work.

One of the most important steps to making your dreams a reality and discovering *Your Action Potential* is choosing something you love and finding a way to incorporate it into your daily life. That may mean quitting your comfy (but boring) desk job for something more "you." Now, that doesn't mean you should be irresponsible here. It just means that you should take the time to figure out what you love and how you can make a living doing just that!

For instance, I know a writer who dreamed of spending her days writing books. Yet she toiled away at a public relations job to pay the bills, certain that no one could make a real living writing. After all, all of the experts said it couldn't be done except by a favored few. Well, after hitting a major life crisis, she discovered a way to write and pay the bills—plus she can stay home with her kids, to boot! My friend now ghostwrites books for other authors and professionals and publishing houses. Gone are the days of writing stuff she hates. Now she chooses her clients and her projects and has the flexibility to say no when she wants to take the kids away for a few days of vacation or play in the snow on a cold winter's morning.

Sure, she loves when the opportunity arises when she can see her own name on the jacket of a book. But ghostwriting allows her to do what she loves and make the money she needs to pay the mortgage. And that's what it's all about: fulfilling your passion and attaining your dreams despite what others think or say!

So, what do you *really* want to do with your days and your life? Take this opportunity to really think about what you'd love to do day in and day out. You can't imagine how exhilarating, not to mention freeing, it is to jump out of bed each morning anxious to get to work! Don't waste another day at a dead end job that drains the energy from your body and your life. Make a commitment right now to find something you love, and go for it!

Sidebar:

Discovering Your Passion
True happiness comes when you do what you are most passionate about. But how do you uncover your passion? The clues are all around you. Here are a few tips to get your started:

Step One: Get quiet. How can you even attempt to realize your passion if you don't even know yourself? Take the time to slow down, reconnect with yourself in a whole new way, and engage in activities you enjoy. You'll be surprised at how quickly your true passions begin to emerge.

Step Two: Become sensitive to your environment. Take notice of what's going on around you and how those things (and people) make you feel. Read the newspaper more carefully. What stories fuel your fire? Those are the things and topics that you are most passionate about. Now, how can you use this newfound knowledge to discover what will make you happiest in life?

Step Three: Answer a series of questions. Next, ask yourself these simple questions:

- What interest or desire am I most afraid to admit to myself and others?
- What do I love most about myself?
- What have I always dreamed of doing?
- What special thing have I always put off doing?
- What could I do to make the world a better place?

Step Four: Go hunting. Look around your home. What things excite you most? Do you love pictures? Why not take up photography? The things that make you feel the most love are connected to your passion. Now it's your job to figure out how.

Step Five: Take a risk. Stop thinking about your passions and start doing something. Take a risk and step out to try something new.

Fine-Tune Your Greatest Asset: You!

Want to succeed in life? Want to discover your full *Action Potential?* Then you must make yourself the best you that you can. Now, that doesn't mean turning yourself into a well-buffed supermodel. If I could show you how to do that, I'd have a lot more books on the shelf bearing my name. What I'm talking about here is accepting the fact that the way you look and present yourself in and to the world really will have an impact on what you are able to accomplish.

It never ceases to amaze me how many people come out of college sporting modern body piercing, tattoos, and off-the-wall hairstyles and coloring and don't expect that it will affect their job interview for a teaching job, a receptionist's spot, or even a marketing position at a high quality company. Should what we look like effect our ability to get a good job? No, it shouldn't, if we're qualified. Does it? Absolutely!

Now, I know that this may seem a bit contradictory, especially since we have been discussing forging your own way and stepping beyond what's considered "normal" to achieve your dreams. But when it comes to your outward appearance and attitude, conforming is sometimes just what is required.

Does this mean that to become successful you must wear a pin-striped suit and keep your hair cut to exactly one inch above your collar? Not in the least. What it does mean is that you must appear appealing in a non-threatening manner. That includes making yourself into the most amazing you that you can be.

Keep this in mind: no matter what you do, you will never appeal to everyone. The key here is to make the law of attraction work for you, not against you.

So, what is this law of attraction that everyone is talking about? Simply put, it is a philosophy that states that you are a living, breathing, life-sized magnet. It's up to you and your thoughts what you allow your magnet to attract—good things or bad. Any thoughts you have (positive, negative, happy, sad, etc) will grab hold of similar thoughts. So, if you extend warmth to the world, you'll get warmth back; but if you extend frustration and meanness to the world around you, that's what you'll also experience.

What does this mean? Put anything but your best out there and you'll get less than the best back. Starting to get it now? By following the law of attraction, you will be able to better see yourself (and others) for who they really are, and command more good things for yourself in the process.

Now let us get back to putting your own best foot forward. Let's say that your clothes are rumpled, your hair is tangled, and you forgot to take a shower before heading out to that big job interview. You know that you are by far the most qualified candidate. You're good at what you do, and your resume proves it! The guy sitting next to you has half of the experience, virtually no training, but he's dressed in a professional manner and presents himself well. Who do you think is going to get the job? The odds are the other guy is. Why? Because he put out his very best. Even though his best was lacking in some areas, it was still his best, and he reaped the rewards. That is the law of attraction at work.

So, where do you start in order to make this law of attraction thing work for you too? Let's begin with our basic senses.

The Sense of Smell

Like it or not, one surefire way to attract or repel someone is the sense of smell. Strong odors are usually discouraged since they have the tendency to turn people off—even when they are good smells. Bad breath and body odor has the tendency to attract negativity no matter what the situation. First impressions do count, and oftentimes smell is the first, most important impression that you can make.

Appearance

The way you look can also have a lot to do with your ability to generate success. More complex than the smell issue (after all, if you smell bad, you smell bad), appearance can be a very subjective thing. What one person considers inappropriate, another may consider individualism. That said, let's talk about the basics.

In the business world, there are a few things that are considered "musts" in regard to appearance:

- Your clothes must be neat and clean. Keep in mind, that it is not the cost of your clothing that counts, it's the look you are after. Your clothing should (and must) fit into whatever role you are trying to portray. After all, a doctor in an emergency room isn't going to show up for work in a skin-tight cocktail dress and stiletto heals, is she? By comparison, a prostitute sporting a conservative, Amish-looking getup probably isn't going to drum up much business. Look the part, whatever that part may be. Otherwise, you risk not being taken seriously for who and what you and your job are. Not sure what look you should be after? Ask for help. Look for people who fit the role you're after, and ask them to help you choose a few good outfits. Or head to the store and find a salesperson that looks the way you want and need to look. They'll be happy to get you started—especially if they work on commission! Remember this, though: never go so far out of your comfort zone that you feel uncomfortable or silly. Confidence will give you an edge. Dressing for success requires dressing with confidence, and if you're constantly pulling at your collar or fidgeting with your skirt, then you will appear less confident. In this case, find a compromise between your current look and the so-called norm.

- You must sport a well-groomed look. I know, I know—your hair and makeup is who you are. You love those purple stripes and can't for the life of you figure out how they affect the way you work. Or you're a guy who likes a little length to his locks and his look. The fact remains that in some businesses and industries, a more conservative look will yield better results. I recommend finding a well-groomed, neat look that fits both the office and your lifestyle. If you are a male, remain clean-shaven, or at least be sure that any facial hair you sport is carefully groomed. Both sexes should work hard to keep their skin as clean and clear as possible, even if that means hitting the salon for some advice and maintenance. Yes, guys, I mean you too!

- You must appear confident. The fact is, no one will ever feel like they are perfect. You will always notice a wrinkle in your shirt, a bulge in your belly, or some other negative aspect to yourself or your appearance. That doesn't have to hold you back. Those lacking confidence in themselves and their abilities rarely succeed. Why? Because no one can be sure they have what it takes to make it to the top—whatever that top may be. The point I'm trying to make is to continue to work toward becoming your best, even when you feel like you are falling short—way short. Look the best you can today, and maximize its effects. Do the same tomorrow and the next day and the next, and you are bound to improve the way you look and feel about yourself.

Confidence is a million-dollar word. It is something that happens when you have all of the other issues discussed, ironed out, and working in an efficient manner. It is the most attractive quality for any man or woman to possess. One thing we should address here: there is a huge difference between being *confident* and being *cocky*. Cocky means being overly self-confident or self-assertive; while confident means being full of conviction and having or showing assurance and self-reliance.

Take a look at those two definitions. You will immediately see why you would want to be called confident and not cocky. One is positive; the other negative. One describes someone who is truly good and understands who they are, while the other does not.

Sidebar:

Confidence Boosters

Need a few simple ways to build your confidence? Here are a few basic confidence boosters to give a try.

Sometimes, you don't have time for a long formula or to sit down and work through a process. There are times where you need confidence fast—instant confidence. Here are five ways to get an instant boost of confidence.

1. Look for compliments.
   Be on the lookout for them. They reveal the value others see in you.

2. Log your successes.
   Whether it's the first webpage you completed, first song you played on the piano, or the first million you made in business, keep an ongoing list of your own personal success stories.

3. Acknowledge your abilities.
   What great skills and talents do you possess? Keep an "I'm good at" list to help remind you what you can do well, for those times when everything seems to be going wrong.

4. Find support.
   Have someone in your life who believes that all your crazy dreams can come true? Good! It can be good to have someone on your team who isn't based in "reality." Or, if that's not an option, seek constructive feedback from peers you trust. Those who give constructive feedback boost your confidence by showing you what's right and helping you improve what's wrong.

Action Potential Exercise

When it comes to bringing out the very best you that you can, I have found this exercise very helpful.

First, find a quiet place where you will not be disturbed for at least thirty to sixty minutes. I know, to many of you this may seem like an impossibility, but it is essential; so find a way to make it happen. Take every bit of external stimuli and get rid of it. That means the phone, people, and the television set—anything that may disturb you even for a split second, especially that ticking clock hanging on the wall.

Once you have found this quiet place, clear your mind, focusing on just you and your breathing. Once you've been able to clear your mind of all thoughts (this may take a few minutes), you will be ready for the next step, called visualization.

Sit in total silence. Stay focused. Now, concentrate on all of the traits that you believe a confident person would possess. Next, pretend in your mind that you already possess each of these qualities. This is the scientific term of "faking it until you believe it and make it true."

Why is this exercise important? Because until you can possess the main trait of confidence (believing in yourself and your abilities), you can't move forward on your quest.

This exercise is most effective when performed several times a day until this new reality is true to you. Then, and only then, will you begin to experience a real change in yourself and reap the rewards of true confidence.

Now that you fully understand the true components of fine-tuning your greatest asset—you—use it, and accelerate yourself to the next level of awareness.

Mind Over Matter: Using Yours to Succeed!

Consider this: "Everything that happens in life is your responsibility and where you are right now is exactly where you need to be. It suits you."

Now, before you close this book for good, let me explain. The above phrase makes two things absolutely true:

1. No one is a victim. It is what you do with a situation that makes you a victor.

2. Until you accept responsibility for what's happening in your life (even the adversity), you cannot learn from it in order to create a better outcome.

Have you ever talked to someone who insists that they just have bad luck? Can you think of someone who always gets close to their goals, only to have them derailed before completion? Are you that someone? Maybe you're letting your mind take over and thwart your success.

As we've already discussed, our inner voice is jam packed with a database full of negative comments that we've both heard and told ourselves. This can lead us to sabotage our own efforts for success by limiting our ability to believe in ourselves enough to even try something new.

Then there are those of you who have enough confidence to try, yet you can't seem to finish anything. These are the people who always let something happen to stop them in their tracks. I contend that these "somethings" aren't the result of bad luck, or even a lack of desire and ability. They are a direct result of your inability to allow yourself to move forward. The mind is a powerful thing, and you are letting yours take over and stop your heart and your passion from taking you where you really want to be. It's time to take back control of your mind and teach it to work for you, not against you.

Let's get back to that person who "something always happens to." This person is obviously not letting their mind work with them. It's like a tug-of-war, with their heart saying, "I want to get a better job," and their mind stopping their progress by telling them they aren't savvy enough to say the right things at their interview, so why bother even showing up?

So, what do people like this do to stop sabotaging their lives? First they need to recognize what they're doing. Then they have to evaluate when they are most likely to sabotage their own efforts and how they do it. For instance, maybe you are the type of person who has great aspirations, but no gumption to actually get anything started; or maybe you get new projects started all right, but always find a reason to quit before you ever finish and succeed. The fact is you can't get away from yourself, so you'd better find a way to work with yourself for your best interests.

Once you are able to identify your triggers (what sets you on that downward spiral), you'll have a better chance at changing those behaviors for better ones. This isn't going to be easy. As a matter of fact, it's probably going to be very hard. The key is to recognize those old behaviors, stop them right away, and substitute new behaviors that better suit you. You'll love the way you feel once you dig in your heels, finish what you start, and experience true success in doing it.

Here's something to ponder: most rewards come at the end of a project. If you've never let yourself finish something important, you have no idea how great the reward can be. Think about that the next time you are about to sabotage your own best efforts.

Sidebar:

Action Potential Exercise

Every situation that happens to you in your life presents a challenge to overcome and learn from. That's what makes us each stronger, smarter, and more capable to handle what else may come our way.

You don't want to be one of those people who are

always feeling sorry for themselves. This is the road to nowhere, and hey, you're headed somewhere! The simple fact is we learn more from experiencing pain than we do from experiencing pleasure. Embrace this truth the next time a painful situation rears its ugly head.

When you look at adversity as a learning experience, there will always be a positive outcome. Life is about learning and growing. Now, let the growing continue!

Programming Yourself to Succeed

Why do we let other people influence the way we think about ourselves and our abilities? Worse yet, why do we sometimes treat ourselves so badly, telling ourselves that we aren't good enough, handsome enough, smart enough, etc? It's all in the way we have been programmed.

Programming is something you do to a computer, right? Well, your brain is one big computer, and it has been being programmed since your first breath. Other people help program it, and so do we by the things we tell ourselves.

The amazing thing is we tend to believe whatever is being programmed into us, even the bad stuff. Why? Because our brain simply can't fathom the fact that we would tell ourselves something that wasn't true.

Now, this can be an amazing gift if our parents took

the time and energy to program only good thoughts into our brain. When this happens, we tend to follow their lead and do the same with our own internal programming thoughts.

When, however, our parents weren't able to properly program our growing brains, we began to believe all of "the junk" and feed more and more of it into ourselves. When this happens, it can be devastating.

Now, we've all heard success stories of children who have overcome great odds and survived abuse and neglect to do great things—or at least live a relatively normal life. How was that possible? Somehow, they figured out how to reprogram their brain in order to get those bad thoughts out and replace them with good, positive ones. And I'm here to tell you that you can too!

Your subconscious mind is the part of the brain that works below the level of conscious perception. Imagine 1,500 words or more flowing through your mind every minute! Some good, some bad, depending on your programming, of course. Every time you hear "You are—," or you tell yourself "I am ___," those words are being embedded into your subconscious. It doesn't take long to start believing it. After all, it is who you are. Right? It doesn't have to be.

Your Action Plan Exercise #1:

Here's a solution to getting rid of those negative "I" statements we're all famous for. Learn to say a new four-letter word: *stop!* Anytime you catch yourself beginning to say (or think) any type of negative "I" statement, say the word *stop*, then replace what you were about to say with something positive. For example, when you've forgotten something, your initial response may be to say something to yourself like," I can't believe how stupid I was to forget my keys." *Stop!* Instead, say "I certainly won't forget my keys next time now that I know what trouble it causes."

Don't be surprised if you find yourself saying *stop* quite a lot when you begin using this technique. It takes practice to learn to speak kindly to yourself. But it's important. Your brain wants to believe everything you tell it, so you'd better be sure to only tell it good things (especially about yourself!).

Don't Forget, You're In Control

There is a huge secret that I'd like to share with each of my readers, because I think it is so important: the secret is that you are the *only* person in the entire world who can let someone affect your conscious and subconscious mind. That's an empowering thought, isn't it? Yet, it's so true.

Think about a time when someone has hurt your feelings. They couldn't have done it if you didn't let them. You have the power to control your own feelings and destiny. Don't give that power to anyone else! Be the gatekeeper who decides whose opinion matters and whose doesn't! How? First, by deciding that your own opinion matters, then deciding who you'll listen to and who you won't. It really is that simple.

Your Action Plan Exercise # 2:

Whenever someone tries to instill their negative opinion on you and you don't want to accept it, simply say, "I'm sorry you feel this way." This allows both parties to move on their way without affecting the other person. It is not offensive to basically disagree with their feelings in a way that does negatively impact your own. It does allow both of you to be heard and neither to take responsibility for the others' feelings.

Once again, you've discovered another step to creating a blueprint to *Your Action Plan*. Using these tips, neither you, nor anyone else, will be able to get in the way of you building your subconscious or conscious mind; unless, of course, you allow it.

Remember, these parts of your mind are the very building blocks that your whole life is built with. Keep them safe. Your life depends on it!

The Power of Money

Money causes more trouble than anything else on earth: divorce, war, hatred, insecurity, crime—you name it, money is the root cause. In contrast, it also creates a lot of wonderful and good things: security, beauty, art, love, and more.

Money isn't evil; but "people can be evil when it comes to money." It's the way we view money and use money that causes all the trouble. When we let our happiness and our lives depend on the amount of money in (or absent from) our wallets, trouble is bound to ensue.

With this in mind, remember:

1. Money does not bring happiness!

2. Money does not solve all of your problems! They're here to stay until you figure out a solution.

3. Money will not make your relationship better.

Think I'm wrong about these points? Think about a group of newlyweds from the past (maybe yourself included). Newly married couples rarely have any money (especially the young ones). They must work together to build a nest egg, careers, and a family. It's a struggle to be sure, but most of the time they are happy just to have each other. Now fast forward ten or even twenty years. The house is bigger, the cars are better, and the bank account is larger. Is the couple happier? The answer is usually no, they are not. More often than not, they are unhappier now than in any other time in their marriage? Why, because the stresses of life and money have taken a toll on their lives, their energy, and sometimes even their love. The things we do with money can make us feel safe and happy, or can destroy everything we hold dear. This is up to us and the relationship we have with it.

Here's another important reason to come to grips with how you view money: when you do not have a good working relationship with money, you will never be financially stable. Again, you scoff at my insight. *Sure, he can say that*, you think. *He's a doctor; he has money.*

Let's think about it. How many people do you know that have great jobs that pay them handsomely, yet they are always on the brink of despair? Maybe they've bought too big a house; or their kids go to a school beyond their reach; it doesn't matter what they spend their money on, the point is they spend it and then some.

Now, take the guy working at your local gym. He

can't make much. Chances are he makes in a week what you make in a day. Yet, he's always smiling, never seems to worry about the clunker sitting in the parking lot with his name on the title. He has what he can afford, and he's content with that. This guy makes virtually nothing, yet he is more financially stable than the guy with the Jaguar and six-bedroom house featured above. Why? Because the second man knows what money *is* and what it *isn't*. It is the means by which we can take care of our needs (and a few wants along the way); it isn't something to be used for power, prestige or to make us feel better about ourselves.

Money is powerful. The question is: what kind of power do you want it to have over your life?

Money as Energy

Money is an energy source; nothing more, nothing less. It allows us all to do the things we want in life. Certainly, money allows us all the opportunity to "afford" to do the things we want to do: go on nice vacations, eat out, have nice clothes, etc. And there's nothing wrong with enjoying it. Problems arise, however, when money begins to rule our lives. Money in itself is not bad, unless you will do anything to get more of it. When, however, you begin to use it for a greater good, then your relationship with money will improve, and believe it or not you will be more content with less, thereby eliminating the stress of needing more and more.

By now, some of you are beginning to feel a little perturbed. *What does he know?* you may be asking yourself. *He doesn't live my life and have to pay my bills.* I agree we all need money to survive. It puts food on our table and a roof over our heads. My goal right now is to simply get you to look at money a little differently and put some real attention on it—positive attention, that is it! By doing this, you'll have a better idea of what your relationship with money really is and how much you really want and need.

The simple truth is you can make as much money as you want. It's up to you. But you can't make that amount if you don't know what it is. Sound impossible? It really isn't. Most financially successful people decide early in their careers what type of salaries they want and find a job or career that fits within their interests that will make that amount of money. You can too!

Now, let's discuss some seldom looked-at laws regarding money.

Law #1: Those who think govern those who work.

Think about it. Those who are in the highest paid occupations are usually those who use their brain for a living, not their muscle. It isn't the laborer or the road worker bringing in hundreds of thousands a year, despite their long hours of demanding physical work. It's the engineer who designed the road they are building or the architect who designed the skyscraper they are working on.

The energy used to plan and design will always have a greater effect than physical ability alone. Now, don't let this confuse you into thinking that you won't have to work hard for your money. These thinkers work very hard—they just use more brain power than muscle power.

Law #2: We have to create value.

In order to receive money, people need to feel as if they are taking in more than they are giving out. This is what we call perceived value. If your product is "X," then your customer must feel as if they are getting "X" plus ten in order to feel they are getting a real value. Sound like a simple idea? It is. That's what sales are based on.

Oh, but you say you don't like sales. Get over it. Everything in your life revolves around sales in one way or another. It's a learned response we begin using at the earliest of ages. Take my young nephew, for instance. He must have only been three or four when I took him to the grocery store to pick up a few things. Seeing a display for his favorite cookies, he began his "sales pitch" through the store. "But we have some at home," I assured him. "We'll get some as soon as we get back." That wasn't good enough. He proceeded to explain to me how there might not be enough for both of us (and he didn't want me to miss out on having any), they might not be any good (after all, they've been in the cupboard awhile), or someone else may have already eaten them (and he certainly didn't want to inconvenience me with a trip back to the store). The little salesman was on a roll.

Do you think anyone taught him these techniques? Certainly not. I honestly believed that both of our lives would be better if we bought a new pack of Oreos, and he let me know that in no uncertain terms.

We use those same techniques to get what we want in life. We smile, we cajole, we demand. We do whatever is necessary to get our own "new pack of cookies" by showing the other person its value.

Law # 3: Always give joyfully.

I'm sure that you have heard this time and time again: a joyful giver is paid back tenfold. The universe is very good at reciprocating, especially when you joyfully give of your time, your talents, and your money. Now, that doesn't mean that you should give with the express purpose of getting back. The universe is also very good at seeing through this smokescreen. It rewards honest intent, and motivation, not manipulating ones. Give to give. It'll make you happy and give the universe a reason to smile upon you too.

Law # 4: Be willing to accept money.

It may be hard to believe, but yes, some people actually have a hard time accepting money. They stay at a poor-paying job because they don't feel that they deserve a better paying one. They price their home below market value because they don't have enough confidence that the work they've completed on it is worth much. After all, they did it themselves; how good could it really be?

I see this defeatist attitude all of the time, and it breaks my heart. These poor people allow themselves to struggle financially when they really don't have to.

The simple fact is it's impossible to acquire wealth if you will not accept money. From now on, you will accept money with ease. Why? Because you know that you deserve it. Want a raise? Ask for one! Who's going to offer you a thirty percent salary increase when they don't have to? If you've never balked at three percent, then the company loses out to offer you more—even if you are worth it. But before you do that, find out what you're worth. The answer may surprise you.

Now, sit down and come up with a number. Make sure the number is not too low. Otherwise, resentment will begin to seep in and you will feel taken advantage of. Of course, if you set your value too high, you won't believe in it yourself and will be unable to convince anyone else that you're worth it either. Therefore, pick a number that you can realistically live with.

Now, every step you take toward your goal should be taken in a way that gets you closer to that number. Maybe that means looking for a new employer or changing careers altogether. Or maybe it means starting your own business. That's up to you. The point is to find a way to get what you're worth.

Law # 5: Make sure that "it" is not about the money.

What is "it?"

"It" refers to doing what you are doing only for the

sake of the money. That is why in previous chapters I asked you to find something that you love, and find a way to make the kind of money you want doing that. When "it" is about money, "it" will never work. The laws of the universe first want us to do good things, and then be compensated for it. Not to do whatever to make the most we can. Does that make sense?

My personal thought is that no amount of money will ever be enough. There will always be new ways to spend it, and spend it we do! So why stop working so hard to have the next best thing when we can be perfectly happy with what we have right here and right now, if only we would let ourselves.

I remember speaking to a woman once who said she couldn't think of a single thing to ask for Christmas because she literally had everything she wanted and needed. Now, you might think this woman was dripping in fur coats and jewels. But she was just an average, ordinary woman I drummed up a conversation with in the dentist's office. Her pitch to me was that sure, there lots of thing to want, but nothing she really needed. What an awesome way to live! The money she had was more than enough. Why? Because at some point she made a conscious decision that she decided didn't even need that much!

To get satisfaction from what you do, it cannot be about money. I learned that early on in my medical career. I was in a doctorate program in the final year of clinic when a very successful doctor came into our class to give a seminar on how to build a successful practice.

His main secret, he told us, was making the patient believe that you cared about them. Then he proceeded to show us how.

This was his secret? I wondered. Maybe it was the way he phrased it, or how I received it, but it didn't sit well with me. I raised my hand and said, "The doctor said that you should pretend and make them believe you really care. Even if you don't."

There was an odd pause, then the doctor retorted, "Yes, and how do you do that?"

My answer remained the same: "Just care for them in the same way that you would like to be cared for if you were ill."

The reaction I received from my other classmates, as well as the visiting speaker, made me realize a startling fact that day: not everyone shared my philosophy. Some of them didn't care one iota about being a caregiver or a healer. They were in it for the money. How sad to think they have spent their lives doing something without any passion or drive. I venture to say many of them probably live miserable, stress-filled lives that no amount of money can remedy.

Find a way to help people (including yourself) thrive instead of survive, and you will be fulfilling more than a quest to make more money. You will have found a true calling that will more than likely compensate you handsomely for your efforts. Never fall for the same promise of the big bucks as my fellow students. It will only sustain you for a short period of time.

Remember these words by BJ Palmer: "You *make a living by what you get. You make a life by what you give.*"

Law # 6: "It" comes from other people.

This is the ultimate law, which is why I saved it for last. Now that you have found something that you love and a way to make huge sums of money doing it, you'll need to find a consumer or an audience who's willing to pay you for it. This will require vigilant expansion and growth in order to thrive. Always look for new avenues to expand before your current ones dry up. This theme is hit home in the amazing book, "Who Moved My Cheese" by Spencer Johnson. In short the characters in the book, who happen to be mice, were looking for their cheese and somehow it wasn't there anymore. The smart one found new cheese before he had to and lived a happy life. The others weren't so fortunate. I won't spoil the rest of the book for you. The point is to always be looking for new progressive things to do. Do not just be motivated when your other options have dried up.

This chapter has started you off on a new relationship with money. Give it some thought and attention today to build a lasting relationship for the future.

Sidebar:

How do you view money?
There's nothing quite like money to get the juices flowing. It has been the subject of songs, books, and seminars. It seems as if no matter how much you have, you want more. How you view money has a lot to do

with how you make it, spend it, and even live by it (or despite it).

Some people have a lot of money and are afraid to spend a penny, while others have no money and don't really seem to care. Then there's the group that spends every dime they get—quickly.

So what's your view on money? Do you hoard it? Treasure it? Give it away? Don't really think about it? Not too concerned with it? Try to save/build it? For what purpose are you doing these things? You need to figure that out before you can change the way you look at money.

It's time to see money for what it is: a way to get what we want. Decide what that is and the rest will come much easier.

Sidebar:

The Facts about Money

Want to change the way you look at money? Consider some of these quirky facts:

- If you had 10 billion $1 notes and spent one every second of every day, it would require 317 years for you to go broke.

- How long does money last? That depends on the denomination of the note. A $1 bill lasts 18 months; $5 bill, two years; $10 bill, three years; $20 bill, four years; and $50 and $100 bills nine years before they are replaced.

- How much does $1 million weigh? That would depend on the denomination of the bills you use. Since there are 490 notes in a pound, if you used $1 bills, it would weigh 2,040.8 pounds, but if you used $100 bills, it would weigh only 20.4 pounds.

- The Bureau of Engraving and Printing produces 38 million notes a day with a face value of approximately $541 million.

- Almost half (48%) of the notes printed by the Bureau of Engraving and Printing are $1 notes.

- Martha Washington is the only woman whose portrait has appeared on a U.S. currency note. It appeared on the face of the $1 Silver Certificate of 1886 and 1891, and the back of the $1 Silver Certificate of 1896.

Don't Wimp Out!

What are you saying to yourself on a daily basis? Are you offering up a variety of kind, gentle, inspiring words, or just a bunch of negative, self-defeating bunk? Not sure? Try this simple exercise: whenever you're alone, think out loud. I usually avoid doing this when people are around, lest they think I'm a bit crazy.

Listen to what you're saying; I mean, really listen. Do you like what you hear? Would you ever say these things to someone else? If not, then ask yourself this: why are you saying them to yourself? You deserve better!

Tuning into your personal thoughts is the first step in changing the negative self-talk that's been holding you back from more positive inspiration.

But first, let us discuss why we beat ourselves up so with the way we speak to ourselves when no one else is listening. Negative self-talk does serve a purpose. When you're scared of trying something new and you tell yourself, *I can't do that! I'm a stupid fool to even think of it!* You are likely to listen, not give it a try and, sure enough, relive your fear. Maybe that's good in some rare situations, but not if you are trying to grow as a person.

Many people use negative self-talk to protect themselves from failure by actually talking themselves out of things. After all, if you never say hello to that nice-looking woman in the next office, she'll never ask you out and you'll never risk getting hurt (or making a fool of yourself). Unfortunately, guarding yourself to this extent also ensures that you won't experience any of the good things that could also happen.

The trouble with negative thinking is that it all-too-easily becomes automatic—our first response to everything. And that, my dear reader, can be a real problem.

Negative self-talk can keep you a prisoner to your own limitations. How? Some of the most common ways is by:

- Emphasizing your past failures and making it more difficult to move forward in new situations.

- Ignoring anything good that happens.

- Setting impossible standards of perfection.

- Assuming others' thoughts about you are negative.

In the end, all of these things are your way of insuring that your never reach *Your Action Potential.*

Now, let's get practical here. Would you accept

someone calling you a jerk? Of course not! That's inappropriate, not to mention mean. So, why do you say that and worse to yourself? Now, come on, admit it. We've all been caught doing it.

Okay, so maybe you aren't quite so mean (or vivid) about it. Maybe your negative self- talk is a bit more subtle, like making excuses for why you can't (or shouldn't) go for that promotion, start up a conversation with someone new, or basically anything else that you're avoiding.

In order to break this destructive cycle, it's important to take command of your speech. Look for words like "if," "can't," and "but." They're all wimpy ways of holding yourself back. Instead, use words like "can" and "should." Instead of constantly talking yourself out of things, talk yourself into them for a change.

The next time your boss is picking people to attend a seminar, don't shy away from putting your name on the list because "you don't do anything important enough around the office to warrant the expense." Instead, think of all of the ways the seminar will help you do a better job, and let your boss know it. You just might find yourself on the next plane to Miami.

Useless Words to Avoid

There are some words that are "stealing" words. They steal our self-confidence and make us think that we deserve less than we really do. So, what are the worst stealing offenders? Here are a few that must be taken out of your vocabulary right now:

Try-The word "try" implies failure. Not good at all. What's a good replacement? "Do." So the next time you notice yourself using "try" in a sentence, rephrase it to something that states when you will accomplish the deed (or do it). You do not try; you either do or don't do. That's the bottom line in every action in life. The rest is up to you.

Can't-The next useless word to toss from your mindset is the word "can't." It has only two possibilities: you either don't know how to do something (which can be remedied), or you don't want to do something (which is totally up to you to change). Once you stop using the word "can't," you will see an automatic increase in your productivity.

But-The last useless word to avoid is the word "but." This is a word that is used as an excuse. It has been proven that every time but is used in a sentence, everything else said before it is considered untrue. So if you say, "I could go to college, but…" what you're really saying is I can't go to college. Now, which did you really want to say? Consider that the next time "but" creeps into your sentence.

So, what can (and should) you replace the word "but" with? Try "and." What this does is allow you to mean both portions of your sentence without creating a negative impact. For instance, when fighting with your spouse, you could say something like, "I love you, and I would like to not argue with you over dinner." This makes everything in the sentence true. You do love that person, and you do not want to fight.

The scary thing about these insidious words is how

they change what you're saying (and how you will react), without you ever really noticing it. Your success in life is directly proportional to your communication with yourself and with others.

Wimpy, negative words no longer have any place in your vocabulary—especially when you're talking to yourself. Get rid of them right now and replace them with some of these instead:

Know-Knowing is the act of confidence and the security to be sure in your ability.

When-When can you get the things you need to get done actually done? When will the project be completed? When can I expect the estimate I asked for? When makes things happen. It requires commitment to answer a when question. Try it; you may be surprised at the outcome.

Challenges-Wouldn't it be nice to never have another problem in life? From this day forward, you don't. You face challenges. By using the word challenge instead of problem, you are telling yourself that what you are facing can be handled and fixed. Problems are far too difficult to remedy. Challenges, on the other hand, can be overcome.

It may seem overly simplistic to change a few words in your vocabulary and expect big change. But remember, everything counts, and small changes can and will have a big impact!

Manifesting

Wouldn't it be nice if all of your thoughts came true? It happens all of the time. The trick is to choose the ones you want to manifest into reality.

Have you ever been walking along, seen a bump in the sidewalk and said to yourself, *Don't trip*. What happened next? Chances are you tripped. The reason, of course, is because by saying "Don't trip," you just told your mind that you were going to trip. Now, wouldn't it be great if you could use this unique power to actually accomplish more in life? Now you can!

Any statement with "I" or "I am" goes directly into your subconscious, making it more important than ever to be conscious of what you are telling yourself. We've already discussed the negative effects that our self-talk can have on us; now we're going to talk about how we can manifest our thoughts to create more good in our lives.

But before we can begin our lesson on manifesting

your thoughts, we first must discuss another important element to success: *savoring the wanting as much as the having.*

Human beings, by nature, typically are out for the end result in everything they do, with little attention or regard to the actual journey. I would like to challenge that perception. Only looking toward the end cuts the pleasure of the success to a simple moment in time, when you could have been enjoying the entire process. This simple change in thinking can itself increase your pleasure in life one hundred fold.

The next time you find yourself in a tough spot, envision how you will feel once the project is completed. Let yourself feel the exhilaration of completion and success. This exercise alone can take a daunting task; make it exciting, not to mention easier to handle. The end is near, and when you reach it, you'll enjoy it all the more. If , and only if, you let yourself enjoy the process of getting there.

By finding a way to turn a bad situation into a good one, you become more grounded and more able to finish the task at hand. That's a good way to live your life, don't you think?

Now, let us move forward to learning just how to manifest these good thoughts, feelings, and outcomes.

Manifesting starts with thought. This requires you to become hyperaware of your thoughts right away. This can be difficult for some people, but keep at it. You'll get it in no time. The reason for this new awareness is the fact that most of our thoughts are subconscious. Without taking the time and energy to be aware of them, they are free to roam wherever they like—which can be detrimental to your health and your entire being.

If you're the type of person who has always tended to let your brain wander to more negative thoughts, it will be necessary to take those thoughts (which have tended to derail you in the past) and put the train back on the tracks and keep going. I'm going to say that again: if negative thoughts begin to derail you, put the train back on the tracks and *keep going*. You have not failed, you've just been sidetracked. When your mind drifts, allow it to come back, free of penalty. Now, here are the steps necessary to manifest your thoughts into reality:

Have a laser-sharp image of what you want. You need to take the image of what you want and fine-tune it—and every detail of it—for the clearest picture possible.

Make your vision as great as you want it to be. Do not allow your rational, programmed mind to limit you—when you shoot for something higher than you ever imagined, you just might reach it. And even if you fall a bit short, you're still further ahead than you would have been if you hadn't tried at all!

Act as if your wishes and desires have already come true. Success is self-perpetuating. Think something is true, and it's bound to become just that!

You must feel and trust the universe in order for it to give you what you want.

These are the steps you need to continue on your journey. Put them into action right now. But remember this important point: you need to use these steps all of the time, starting right this minute. Strike while the iron is hot and you are passionate about what you are doing. The best results are obtained when you do it now.

While beginning these simple steps, you might want to begin using this other technique to increase your guided outcome and focused intent. The law of attraction states that your mental intention and attitude draw people and circumstances with similar intention and attitude toward you. By now, you should be noticing that the things that you have never thought much about before have a huge weight on our lives. The good part is that you are finally getting the information that you need to right some wrongs and get the life that you always wanted.

If you happen to be a negative person, the fact is you will unfortunately tend to attract negative people. Here's a little test to try to reinforce this concept: find a group (any group) that is negative. Now, divert the conversation to a positive note. Within minutes, you will be perceived as a smart guy (or gal) and be unwanted within the group. Now, to reinforce this concept further, jump right back into those negative doom and gloom thoughts and discussion. Chances are, the group will warm up to you once again and make you feel wanted.

Now, here's my disclaimer: you will begin to notice that you begin doing this type of thing to better yourself. You will begin to attract some friends to you and repel others. This is the cold, hard truth of the natural selection process.

There are really only two outcomes to this process: you can either bring your friends toward enlightenment, or they'll drag you back to where you were before when you were one of them.

The ball is in your court. The question is what are you going to do about it? You can bring them with you or remove yourself from them. People don't like to change. I understand that. Unfortunately, that may mean that some people in your life will be cut loose.

Remember, potential is just that—*potential*. Gone unused, it is *nothing*. You can have all the talents in the world, but if you never put them to good use, they are wasted. Don't let those around you turn you back into Super Glue. Try to turn them into Super Balls instead.

Solution-based Thinking: The Only Kind Allowed

If you want to be more productive and effective, then it's time to consider solution-based thinking. *What is solution-based thinking?* you may be wondering. In its most basic form, it is focusing on the solution and not the problem. Let me elaborate.

A problem-based person is always talking about the problem. They focus all of their attention and energy on the problem, not the solution. All this really accomplishes is sapping your energy and creating even more problems.

Think of a person that you would consider a problem-based thinker. I bet someone popped into your head rather quickly, didn't it? Maybe even several. Now, what is this person (or people) really like? What they look like? What do they smell like? What does their body language say to those around them? Are they the go-to person in a crisis? Think of all the details. Now, how do you feel when you think of this person?

Your body may be reacting in a number of ways. When I think of people like that, I have the urge to run. I feel as if they are literally drawing me into their negativity, and I want to get away as quickly as I can.

Now, when this happens, you have a choice: you can either get away, or you can let this person bring you down. When I was in Georgia for a conference, I was introduced to terminology that has resonated with me ever since. "They are like crabs in a bucket," one speaker explained.

"What does that mean?" you may ask. Well, I'm going to tell you. When crabs are placed in a bucket, they will, under no circumstances, allow their friends to escape. As soon as one of the group begins to climb up the bucket toward freedom, the others pull him back down. If one is going to get cooked and eaten, they all are. Does that sound like the kind of people you want to be around?

Problem thinkers can be like those crabs. They have a need to pull others around them down into their own bucket of gloom and doom. They find nothing wrong with it and don't even care if you bring it to their attention. Their intent is to make sure that you are so miserable that they feel better about their own circumstances. Sad, isn't it?

Everyone needs some sort of benchmark to determine where they stand in life, and the problem-thinkers want you to be their benchmark for misery. Let me be clear here—you must get rid of these life-sucking soul eaters right away.

For some, this may be a challenge since you may have been friends for years or are part of their family.

No matter. They are bringing you down, and you have to make it stop.

Just a little side note here: as you begin to change, this type of person begins to feel uncomfortable, and what do uncomfortable people do? They try to bring you down even further! Why? Because they are afraid that you are going to leave. Then who can they victimize?

Just because you are growing and changing (in good ways, of course), doesn't mean everyone in your life will be happy for you. Your transformation has already started, so be on the lookout for saboteurs.

No Looking Back

The greatest gift you can give yourself—or anyone else, for that matter—is the gift of living in the present. Think about all of the people you know who are living in the past. Are they enjoying where they are right now? Probably not. Instead, they remain stuck in a time when they perceive all was well, even if it wasn't.

I encourage each and every person reading this book to be present in the moment each and every day. Concentrate on all of your senses with each new experience. When you are aware of the sights, sounds, smells, and touch of things, you experience a much deeper appreciation for what you are undergoing. Let's look at eating.

Think of your favorite meal. Now, close your eyes. Let your mind concentrate on the plate. What's its shape? Color? What does the tablecloth look and feel like? Is it soft? Scratchy? Rough? What kind of silver-ware are you using? Now, turn to the food. Is it hot or cold? Are there side dishes or garnishes on the plate? What about the aroma? As you take that first bite, how does it feel in your mouth? You get the idea. Suddenly, this meal takes on a whole new flavor.

Can you imagine being this present in every moment of your life? That is called living life to its fullest. I would highly suggest trying it.

Now that you have an idea of how it is to a solution-based thinker, what are you going to do? Embrace it and put it into action. There is no doubt that your life will be a greater expression of its previous self once you've embraced this new way of thinking.

Remembering the Crabs

Remember those crabs in the bucket? With those in mind, take a good, hard look at the five people that you hang around with the most. Do they bring you up, or do they bring you down? Because you are so pleased with the changes in your own life, you may want to share your experiences with those closest to you.

People are under the misconception that they are going to live forever. Even though we all know that this is a physical impossibility, we still continue to act as if it were true.

How many times have you heard someone say (or said it yourself), "I'll do it tomorrow," or "I'll start saving as soon as I can"? This type of thinking gets you nowhere and will continue to get those around you nowhere unless they change. The time for everything is *now*. Now is always better than later.

The question remains: how are you going to get everything done now? There is a way. It isn't getting everything done right now, it's getting everything done you have to get done right now. Look at your day as a whole and it probably seems pretty overwhelming. Now, begin to chunk it down, and suddenly you can see how to begin crossing things off of that to-do list. Before you know it, everything is finished.

Planning saves more time than you could imagine. Just by taking a few minutes to plan your day, you can increase your effectiveness and give yourself both the time and energy you need to get it all done. With just a few Action Potential shifts, you can gain an immeasurable amount of time.

Let us start with a bit of advice: worst things first. This sounds like an awful strategy at first, but it really works. Your objective is to get things done. How wonderful would it be if you tackled your most challenging things right away in the morning when you were full of energy? Then did the things you enjoyed most, later in the day, when your energy was waning. Plus, you get to end your day on a fun, happy, and easy note. By doing this simple strategy you will create an evenly productive day. You may even notice that you work through the most challangeing chores faster in anticipation of getting to what you really want to do. This paradigm will allow you to turn your life into the most well-oiled, task-oriented machine known to mankind. Imagine that!

Psychoneuroimmunology: The Key to Health and Wellness

Psychoneuroimmunology is a big word, and one you probably haven't heard much about. It may be considered a new branch of science here in the United States, but it has been used in Eastern philosophy for centuries. At its basic core, Psychoneuroimmunology is a law of life that states a patient's mental state influences their health and healing. Now, before you dismiss the idea that you can will yourself sick (or well) without even knowing it, consider how many times you thought "I can't catch the flu this week; I have too much to do." Well, what happens within days? You've got the flu. But it's even more complicated than that.

First coined by Robert Ader, a researcher at the University of Rochester in New York, psychoneuroimmunology stresses the importance of realizing how stress, hostility, and depression can attack our bodies, weaken our immune systems, and leave us open to all kinds of disease.

First, let's discuss how stress affects our bodies. Most of us have heard about the fight or flight response, a mechanism instilled in our very nature in order to protect us from danger.

With our nervous system, this survival mode mechanism is used to help us know when to stand our ground and when to run when faced with a dangerous situation. When the human fight or flight response is activated, many things begin to happen within your body, including:

- an acceleration of the heart and lungs
- an inhibition of stomach and intestinal action
- the constriction of blood vessels in many parts of the body
- a liberation of nutrients for muscular action
- the dilation of blood vessels for muscles
- an inhibition of lachrymal glands for tear production and salivation
- pupil dilation
- relaxation of the bladder

These are all reactions of our body that we should be thankful for. Without them, we would be in grave danger since we would be left without any clues that we were in danger and could easily fall prey to a number of predators.

The amazing thing about these reactions is that they

happen in a fraction of a second. While amazing and useful when used properly, these same life-saving reactions can become life-threatening if they are enacted on a regular basis with no real need.

When we experience continual stress, causing our fight or flight response to kick in, the natural responses designed to save us begins to play havoc on our immune system, setting us up for illness and disease. As a matter of fact, when we look at disease in association with this fight or flight response, we soon discover that all the major killers in the United Sates are clearly a product of our systems going into overdrive and actually damaging—or at least being unable to help—itself.

Since our nervous system cannot differentiate a real danger from a perceived one, it tends to react in the same manner whether you are being mugged or just trying to get through a bad traffic jam. The only difference is the amount of time each response is supposed to last.

Your Heart and Lungs

Let's take a closer look at how this natural response affects our hearts and lungs. When faced with a danger, our heart and lungs begin to accelerate, forcing more blood and oxygen to our muscular system in preparation for a big exit.

Have you ever heard of too much of a good thing? When your heart and lungs are continually told to increase their output in order to prepare the rest of the body to "run," it increases your blood pressure.

Long-term high blood pressure will ultimately cause some serious health effects, including heart attack and stroke.

The lungs too can be affected negatively by the constant stress of overuse, causing COPD—chronic obstructive pulmonary disease.

You get the idea. When you drive a car, you probably know its maximum capabilities, but if you only ever run it to capacity without regular rest and maintenance, it will surely develop some serious issues. Your body is no different. It has been designed to run at several different speeds and levels. To consistently run in at capacity is only asking for trouble. Yet, most of us try—until it breaks down.

Your Immune System

Few people ever consider that an increased level of stress (thus engaging your fight or flight response) is linked to a decrease in your immune system function. The simple fact is without a healthy immune system that works at peak capacity, you cannot have any real quality of life.

I am always amazed at how little attention people give their immune systems—the one part of their body which protects them from all other invaders.

To help you better understand the detrimental effects stress can have on your immune system, let's take a closer look on how it all works. In order to keep your body's survival functions going, your body makes a chemical called cortisol, which in essence strips the immune system of energy when dispersed in large amounts. When your body decides to continually pump cortisol through your body, it weakens your immune system to the point that once the stress is over, it is unable to fight off other invaders like illness and disease.

A great example of this is when an entire office or school is wracked with a flu epidemic. Inevitably, there will be a few hearty souls who can fight it off and never succumb to its effects. Why? After all, they are subject to the exact same invader as everyone else, yet their immune system is able to fight it off. For whatever reason, their immune system is stronger. And that may have a lot to do with their ability to handle stress better than those around them.

Consider this: when you vomit, is your body sick or well? How about when you have diarrhea? Or have a fever? Most of us assume when these things happen, their body is sick. I'd argue that this is the reaction of a healthy body dealing properly with sickness. Although it may seem easier to reach for a medication to stop these adverse reactions from continuing, keep in mind that they are reactions that are necessary to helping your body ward off whatever is attacking your body, and by stopping the reaction you may actually inhibit healing, causing you to feel sicker for a longer period of time. The longer it takes your body to fight off illness, the more prone you are to catching something else down the line.

Still not convinced? Think of it this way: when you are hungry, what do you reach for? Food, of course.

How about when you are thirsty? Water is great. But what do you reach for when you have a headache? If you said Tylenol, Advil, or some other such pain reliever, you would be *wrong*! The odds are your headache is caused by something else. While alleviating this painful symptom isn't wrong, per se, you should be wary of masking this important sign of illness when you don't know what's causing it. Popping a few pills to forget about it is only going to make things and you worse.

Here's one last analogy to prove my point: when you have a flat tire, you obviously take the time to change it, right? You don't just turn up your radio and keep on driving. So why would you take a pain reliever, a fever reducer, or some other medication to dull an important signal your body is sending you without actually fixing what's wrong?

Our bodies have many built-in systems to protect it from harm. Only under severe circumstances does it turn on itself and use those systems to do harm. A real danger arises when we don't listen to our bodies and take heed of what it's trying to tell us. And that's what psychoneuroimmunology is all about: using what you know about your body and how it works to help it work for you, not against you!

Feeding Your Body

Reaching *Your Action Potential* isn't just about your conscious and subconscious mind and using your thoughts to accomplish your goals. Attaining real health also requires taking a good, hard look at the way you're treating your body and changing those bad, unhealthy habits.

Your Glycemic Index
Obesity is at an all-time high. Despite the negative effects of being overweight has on the way we look and feel about ourselves. It can have a very detrimental effect on our overall health.

One way to battle the bulge (and eat smarter) is to better understand your personal glycemic index and the way the foods you eat may ultimately affect your blood glucose levels—not to mention the way you feel.

When you eat high glycemic foods such as breads, pastas, rice, cereal, and baked goods—you know, all the really good stuff—your blood sugar levels rise quickly. The trouble is these foods can't sustain this high energy level, causing your blood glucose levels to dip sharply in short order.

This can cause a myriad of symptoms such as headaches, dizziness, shakiness, not to mention weight gain since your body craves more sugar to help qualm these symptoms.

Eating lower-sugar foods such as fresh fruits, veggies, whole grains, and legumes can all help to stabilize your blood sugar levels—and your appetite—keeping you from hitting the cookie jar an hour after indulging in a bagel.

That said, have you ever known someone who dropped little (if any) weight after going on a low-glycemic diet? For some, the effects may be minimized by the foods they eat along with the low-glycemic ones, how the food was prepared, and even how their individual metabolism reacts to the foods you eat.

Although some researchers dispute the validity of using a low-glycemic diet as a weight loss option, most agree it is a healthier way to eat and can help most people maintain a healthier weight.

Whole Foods vs. Processed Foods

Food certainly isn't what it used to be. When once we were assured that the foods we bought and used were free of hormones, pesticides, and a number of other additives, today it's considered a bit "kooky" to go out of your way to stay on a preservative free diet. Yet, the fact remains, whole foods are and always will be better for you than processed foods.

While processed foods may be easier and quicker to prepare—not to mention cheaper—they do contain many hidden dangers we would all normally consider fine, including:

Salts. Common table salt is made by refining rock salt, which strips its natural mineral balance, reducing it to ninety-nine percent sodium chloride. What makes up the rest of salt? Additives such as bleaching and free-flowing agents, stabilizers, and aluminum compounds. Even sea salt, if it's white and free-flowing, has been highly refined and is lacking in essential minerals and trace elements. Both contain no nutrients and can be harmful to your health over time.

So, how do you know if you're getting unrefined salt? Whole, unrefined sea salt is light grey, not white! It's also lumpy. Unprocessed salt contains more than eighty essential minerals and trace elements that closely resemble the constituents of human body fluids—blood, lymph, sweat, and tears are all salty.

Sweeteners. Like refined salt, white sugar has been stripped of all its vitamins, minerals, and trace elements that naturally occur in the whole sugar cane plant. The whole plant contains only fourteen percent sucrose, along with fiber, water, and various other nutrients, but the refining process separates the sugar from the molasses (the nutrient-rich part of the sugar plant) making refined, white sugar pure sucrose.

Diets high in refined sugar promote blood sugar imbalances, including hypoglycemia and type two diabetes, which is rising at an alarming rate throughout the world.

There are some more natural sweeteners available, however, that can give you the sweetness you crave without the negative effects on your health:

Sucanat and Rapadura are dehydrated sugar cane juices containing the nutrient-rich molasses that refining typically removes.

Date sugar is made from whole, pulverized dates. It is highly nutritious and provides vitamins, minerals, and fiber.

Raw honey offers a natural sweet taste, along with small amounts of protein, vitamins, minerals, and enzymes. Never buy pasteurized honey; its enzymes have been destroyed by heat. Make sure your honey is from a reputable source and does not come from sugar-fed bees.

Maple syrup, barley malt, stevia (an herbal extract of white chrysanthemum), and rice syrup are other whole-food alternatives that can be used in place of refined sugar.

Fats. Believing that hydrogenated fats such as margarine and vegetable shortening were better for us, many people stopped using natural fats such as butter, only to discover years later these artificial fats load the body with trans fatty acids and other unnatural substances that are far worse than the natural fats they are intended to replace.

Eating whole foods doesn't mean depriving yourself of fats. It means choosing the right fats: natural, unrefined fats which provide your body energy and play an important role in metabolism and in protecting cellular health.

What are the healthiest fats to use? Organic butter from pasture-fed cows and extra-virgin olive oil have been found to be the safest. Cold-pressed, unrefined vegetable oils such as flax seed, sesame, sunflower, or safflower oil are also good in salad dressings. These should be kept refrigerated and must never be heated or used in cooking or baking, as they break down quickly when exposed to air, light, and heat.

The more natural and whole the food you eat, the better it is for your health. Despite what the commercials say, there isn't a single food that has been made more nutritious by processing and refining.

Changing Your Taste Buds

One of the hardest things about switching to a healthier eating plan is getting used to the taste of healthier food options. For many of us who have been conditioned to crave ultra-sweet, fatty, and salty foods, the switch to natural can often seem a bit tasteless.

The good news is that our taste buds can easily be reprogrammed to let foods that are good for us taste great. Remember trying to get a picky toddler to eat a new food? The experts all recommended putting the new food on their plates over and over again until they tried it several times. What you were doing was conditioning their taste buds to like it—and you thought it was a waste of time?

Better yet, the opposite is also true. Excluding foods from your diet will leave you with less cravings for that food and give your taste buds a break so that they can be more receptive to new, healthier foods. For example, most people who voluntarily take up vegetarian diets notice they stop craving animal meat after a couple of weeks.

So if you're worried that you won't like any of the good foods in your local health food store, give them a try anyway. After a few tries, you just might hear yourself saying, "Hey, this is good!"

Eat to Live, not Live to Eat

Food should not be feared; it should be enjoyed. And boy do the French know how to enjoy food! They indulge in decadent desserts, savory meats and sauces, wine, and more. Yet, they have low cholesterol, low body fat, and are among some of the healthiest people on earth. How can that be so? Because they've learned how to use food properly. Eating healthy doesn't have to be boring and tasteless. Just ask the French! They manage to eat well—very well—and still stay thin and healthy. Now you can too!

The French have learned the true "art" of eating. It, according to Mireille Guitliano in her bestselling book *French Women Don't Get Fat*, is due in large part to their respect of food. They eat to live, not live to eat, as most Americans do.

To the French, eating is an event. They never grab fast food and seldom rush through any meal or snack.

They take the time to savor each delectable bite and are known to indulge in a few morsels of the richest desserts without stuffing themselves. One or two bites is often enough to satisfy both your hunger and your need for something sweet, according to Guitliano. The French respect that by sharing desserts and refusing to clean their plates when they are full.

If there's one thing we can learn from the French way of eating, it is to stop eating on the run. When you rush through your meals, you do not allow your brain to register that your body is full, causing you to overeat and gain weight and cause a number of digestion problems. Slow down. Take your time to enjoy food again. It really is the healthiest way to eat.

Can changing your eating habits really give you more action potential? Of course it can! Unless your body is running at peak efficiency, it'll use all your energy to ward off everything from the common cold to more serious diseases like cancer—that's energy you won't have to use for the better and more fun things in life—like chasing your dreams. So, don't overlook this all-important step to achieving your goals. Learn to take care of your body and it'll take care of you in so many more ways than you ever thought possible.

Normal Aging—Is It Normal?

How many times have you heard that "It is just normal aging" or "You know you are getting to that age." How about "You know how things are when people are at that age." I am here to point out something. What is normal? Depending on your source, "normal" can be very bad, even deadly. In my opinion, "normal" just means that nothing has been done in order to change the outcome.

Let's look at an example of two people who are thirty-five years of age. One has a good diet and works out several times a week. The other always eats out at fast food restaurants and considers exercise as going to the cabinet and getting the jumbo sized bag of chips. Here is the big question. Which person is normal? If you look at the definition of the word normal, it states, a conforming with, adhering to, or constituting a norm, standard, pattern, level, or type. Now knowing this, the definition of "normal" is an insult and possibly a death sentence. The whole theme of this book is if you are normal and do normal things you get normal results. We both know that isn't what you want, so I am going to tell you how your body ages and how to slow down the "normal" aging process.

There are several systems of our body—eleven to be exact. Each and every one of them has a specific purpose to perform in your body. They perform these specific tasks to allow the body to survive. The body is such a complex piece of machinery that it can have a trillion chemical reaction occurring simultaneously and then do it all again in the next split second. We only have a very limited understanding of the human body. I do know that it is a better idea to work with the body instead of "trick" it or worst yet try to work against it. I am going to give a few scary statistics to make my point. The United States consumes half of all the drugs made in the world. Now if this were the answer why are we such a sick nation? Maybe drugs are not the way to health. Now I am not saying that some drugs or allopathic medicine are not highly effective in crisis care. What I am saying is that they have some practical application in the crisis care and little, if any, in the health model. Here is a little thought that may hit home with you. When you are thirsty it is a lack of what? The answer is water. When you are hungry it is the lack of what? The answer is food. When you have a headache it is a lack of what? The answer is not a pain killer. It is OK to laugh. You get the point. After crisis care is over we need to seek out the root cause and take care of it instead of just masking the bodies' normal responses.

There are eleven systems of the body and we are going to take a look at each of them:

Circulatory- The Circulatory System is the whole body's transport system. It is made up of a group of organs that transfer blood throughout the body. The heart pumps the blood and the arteries and veins transport it, the main function of this system to move nutrients and oxygen around.

Digestive - The Digestive System is made up of organs that digest and transport food. The body uses the broken down food sources for energy, growth and repair. The excess food that is not needed or cannot be digested is turned into waste and eliminated from the body or stored as fat.

Endocrine-The Endocrine System is made up of a group of glands that that produce the body's long distance messengers or hormones. Hormones are the chemicals that control the body functions, such as metabolism, growth and sexual development. The glands include the pituitary, thyroid, parathyroid, adrenal, thymus, pineal. Also the pancreas, ovaries, and testes. They all release hormones directly into the bloodstream (Circulatory System) which transports the hormones to organs and tissues throughout the body.

Immune- The Immune System is our body's defense against infections and diseases. Whenever there is an outside invader, such as a virus or bacteria, our immune system goes to work.

Lymphatic– The Lymphatic System is also a defense system for the body. Its main purpose is to filter out organisms that cause disease, produce white blood cells, and generate disease-fighting antibodies. It also distributes fluids and nutrients in the body and drains excess fluid to prevent swelling.

Muscular– The Muscular System is made up of tissue that is supported on the skeletal system and when they work in conjunction we have movement. The are three types of muscle, skeletal as mentioned above, smooth muscle such as found in the inside of the stomach and intestines, and cardiac muscle that is found in the heart.

*Reproductive-*the Reproductive System gives us the ability to procreate.

*Respiratory-*the Respiratory System brings air into the body and removes carbon dioxide. It includes the nose, mouth, trachea, and lungs.

*Skeletal-*the Skeletal System is made up of bone, ligaments and tendons. It shapes the body and protects the organs from harm.

*Urinary-*The Urinary System eliminates waste from the body in the form of urine.

The last and certainly not least is *the Nervous System-* The Nervous System is made up of the brain, the spinal cord and peripheral nerves. It is the most important system in the body because it is responsible for controlling every other system. It is the reason the brain and spinal chord are encased in bone for protection. The nervous system sends, receives and processes nerve impulses. These nerve impulses tell your muscles and organs what to do and how to respond to the environment.

So now, finally, I can get to the point. All of these systems work in harmony. When there is dis-harmony or dis-ease, we have problems, problems that can go from something as small as a sore throat to something as serious as cancer. The human body is an incredible machine, about which our knowledge is minimal. That being said "What do you do to take care of your machine?" Normal aging is something that occurs when you do not do anything to help slow or even stop the aging process to a great degree. Do I have your attention?

Alternative healing methods are the key in looking and feeling years younger. The challenge is to get people to experience them before they have a problem. It is easier to stay well than to get well when you are sick. I know that sounds a little stupid and it is still true. If we are practicing true health care then why do so many people only go their doctor when they are sick? How is this for an example: in Ancient China the doctors only got paid when their patients were healthy. So with this example it is a more correct statement to call our Health Care System Sick Care System.

Let us focus on a list of "alternative" healing methods. Chiropractic (Neurological Rehabilitation with light therapy), Qui gong, Tong Ren, Massage, Reiki, Yoga and Acupuncture, Nutrition and Fitness Training to name just a few. Every one of these healing modalities was created to slow down the aging process in one way or another. Each modality plays a role in tuning up that machine we were talking about earlier. By combining these therapies, in a very particular way, we are able to have synergistic affect. If you are interested you can go to www.youractionpotential.com to get a greater understanding on this subject.

I know there is a lot of information in this chapter, and I just wanted you to get a general understanding of the amazing thing that we call the human body. I truly believe that without a healthy body you will have a greater challenge to have a healthy mind and vice versa. I hope this sparks your interest to explore the human body further. You only get one in this life you should take care of it.

A Few Final Words

Your life is yours, and it can be anything you want it to be.

Be a *Victor* not a *Victim*.

Be a *Super Ball* not *Super Glue*.

We are on this planet for only a limited time. Make the most of it.

Time is the only thing we can't get back.

It is not the years in your life. It is the life in your years.

Never let anyone define you in a negative light.

Be happy … you deserve it.

You can't control life; you can control how you act toward it.

Let people you care about know as often as you can.

Respect yourself and others … people will follow your lead.

Adopt a "Good for you" attitude instead of a "Must be nice."

Life is great and things can always be worse.

Put your attention on positive things around you and more will happen.

Now you are armed with this information. You are armed with new eyes to look through and see the life that you deserve.

A GIFT FOR YOU!!!!!!!

For taking the first step toward reaching "Your Action Potential" I am going to give you a free gift. Everyone likes gifts, I do, and I am sure you are the same way. Simply go to www.youractionpotential.com/coupon/ and receive your FREE gift. I think everyone should be rewarded for making good decisions.

ONE THING----YOU HAVE TO CLAIM YOUR GIFT NOW. I AM NOT SURE HOW LONG WE CAN KEEP THIS OFFER GOING.

TAKE ACTION AND KEEP MOVING FORWARD.

Yours in Health,
Dr. Jonathan D Yalowchuk

CPSIA information can be obtained at www.ICGtesting.com
Printed in the USA
BVOW01s1454020916

460804BV00001B/1/P